The
GERM FREAK'S
Guide to Outwitting
Colds and Flu

Guerilla Tactics to Keep Yourself
Healthy at Home, at Work
and in the World

Allison Janse
with
Charles Gerba, Ph.D.

ION ✳ SANITIZED FOR YOUR PROTECTION ✳ SANITIZE

approved by
D.R. GERM

Are You a Germ Freak?

❑ Your exit strategy from a public bathroom rivals an NFL playbook.

❑ Your family and friends think Purell is your scent.

❑ You check elevator riders for anyone who is sniffling and opt for the stairs—even though you're going to the top floor.

❑ You turn public bathroom faucets with a piece of tissue.

❑ You avoid buffets that don't have four-foot-long sneeze guard barriers.

❑ You think BYOB means bring your own bathroom hand towels.

❑ You only go to afternoon movies because they're less crowded.

❑ You consider a mask to be appropriate airplane attire.

❑ You trade your number one spot in the express checkout because the cashier says she has a tickle in her throat.

❑ Your neck hairs bristle when someone coughs within earshot.

If you checked three or more of these boxes, congratulations—you're a full-fledged blatant Germ Freak.

If you checked one or two boxes, you're on your way to becoming one of us.

If you didn't check any, there's still hope for you: Read on.

The
GERM FREAK'S
Guide to Outwitting
Colds and Flu

Guerilla Tactics to Keep Yourself
Healthy at Home, at Work
and in the World

**Allison Janse with
Charles Gerba, Ph.D.**

Health Communications, Inc.
Deerfield Beach, Florida

www.bcibooks.com

Library of Congress Cataloging-in-Publication Data
is available from the Library of Congress

Publisher: Health Communications, Inc.
          3201 S.W. 15th Street
          Deerfield Beach, FL 33442-8190

Cover design and inside graphics by Larissa Hise Henoch
Inside design and formatting Lawna Patterson Oldfield

Contents

Part II: The Daily Grime

Part III: Next-Generation Germ Freaks

Germ Freak. (jūrm frēk) *n.* 1 One who is microbe aware. 2 A person cognizant of the power of good and bad germs; one who seeks to avoid and contain the spread of bad germs for his or her personal health and that of others. 3 One who detests being coughed or sneezed on. *Adj.* describing oddly different behavior: "Don't go Germ Freak on me."

> *"Achoo onto others as you would*
> *have them achoo onto you."*
>
> —Germ Freak Creed

Introduction

I wasn't born a Germ Freak. I ate my requisite "pound of dirt before I die" when I was two. My mother was hardly a model of pristine housekeeping. My sisters and I played with dust bunnies the size of desert tumbleweeds, thought spring cleaning meant opening the windows, and until my parents moved from our childhood home, we'd gather in their dining room on holidays and glance at the two-inch hard spot on the rug, fondly remembering our long-deceased dog Heidi who threw up there when I was six. We didn't reap the hygienic benefits of hypoallergenic baby washes; we took consecutive baths in the same water to save money. We didn't have HEPA filters, although my father switched to filtered cigarettes once we were born. And, like most levelheaded mothers, ours preferred spit shine to sanitizer—and we survived.

In college, I shared communal living space without donning flip-flops in the bathroom or worrying whose toothbrush touched mine; I drank from community beer pitchers and shared my first apartment with cockroaches the size of small rats without thinking twice.

Yet two events in my life—two people really—changed my outlook on germs.

The Birth of Triplets:
A Girl, a Boy and a Germ Freak of Nature

My twin daughter and son were born four minutes apart and seven weeks premature. They spent the first two weeks of life in an ICU sporting enough tubes and beeping apparatuses to make any new parent jittery. Upon entering the ICU, Nurse CleanUp Commando led us to a tub-sized basin sink and gave us the hand-washing drill: "Take off any watches and rings and use the scrub brush to remove all dirt from under your nails because it could be dangerous to your newborns' underdeveloped immune system." (*Underdeveloped?*) As I unwrapped the brush from its sterile casing, it occurred to me that I had never given a thought as to what might possibly be growing under my watch or wedding ring, neither of which I had taken off since the previous leap year.

Thankfully, our children had no health issues and were discharged with no dire warnings except to keep them away from "Obviously Sick People."

Once home, my husband and I adjusted to new parenthood as best as you can if neither of you have ever held a baby, much less two at once. Underestimating the number of diapers they'd deplete in a week (*who knew one package wouldn't be enough?!*), I went to the pharmacy to stock up. As I stood in line, I saw the contents of my fellow shopper's basket through sleep-deprived eyes: NyQuil, Vicks Cold and Flu, and three boxes of Kleenex. Just as I was about to move away from this Obviously Sick Person, it happened. I think I felt it the same time I heard it—a big, wet, warm pellet of sneeze. And before I really knew what hit me (literally), another sneeze and a throat clearing that sounded like a seal on steroids. I'd been contaminated! Grabbing the diapers ("No, I don't need my receipt!"), I held my breath all the way to the parking lot and then sucked in as much healthy outside air as I could.

Less than two days later, when I heard the "feed-me" wails times two, I couldn't lift my head from the pillow. It took all the strength I had to sit up, and my reflection in the mirror was a far cry from the glowing moms gracing Pampers ads: I had glands the size of small golf balls, glassy eyes and a face that looked like . . . an Obviously Sick Person. Since my husband had gone to work, I tried to breast-feed my two kids with outstretched arms and inhaled breath. As soon as the babies fell asleep, I scanned the Yellow Pages for a walk-in clinic.

As I sat in the reception area filling out forms, I began the Waiting Room Once-Over: "Sicker than me," "Hypochondriac," "Stay away from him. . . ." One woman directly downwind of me kept coughing and sneezing, trying to nonchalantly inhale a stream of nasal discharge (okay, let's call a snot a snot). She tried to sniff it in to no avail, and then, lacking the energy or courtesy to walk three steps to get a tissue, she wiped her nose with her hand and then wiped her hand on her magazine.

The physician on call prescribed Cipro, a very potent drug noto-
rious for treating anthrax (I now know his choice of antibiotic was
not only wrong but dangerous: See antibiotic resistance page 35).
He told me it was unlikely that my kids would catch what I had,
although he didn't know what I had. He told me to stop breast-
feeding because Cipro can be passed to infants, and assured me I'd
be better in three to five days. Seven days later I still had Titleist
glands. I went to see a throat specialist who prescribed a different
drug, saying that if I got any worse, my tonsils would need to come
out. Luckily, one week later, I was back to near-normal health. Yet
due to one errant sneeze, I spent three weeks in bed, donning a surgical mask and gloves whenever I picked up my kids—hardly the
"mother-child" bonding I'd read was so important. While my husband joked that our children's first view of me would cause them
years of therapy, I wasn't laughing. A Germ Freak was born.

It doesn't matter how or why someone becomes a Germ Freak:
It could be something in your gene pool or the community pool;
it could be innate or something you ate that opened your eyes.
But once it happens, you're forever changed: When others see an
all-you-can-eat buffet and dive in, you see double-dippers help-
ing themselves to an unrefrigerated seafood salad and order off
the menu; when others spy their potential soul mate at a happy
hour, you notice his pale complexion and move on to Bachelor
Number Two. You don't live in a bubble, but you do live with a
heightened sense of awareness. Like a psychic sees auras, you see
someone's germ potential. Like a dog with acute hearing, your

ears perk up when someone sneezes ten cubicles away.

While you'd think you'd be proud of this "sick-sense," many of us are in denial. Some Germ Freaks denounce the "Germ Freak" label, yet freely admit to blatant Germ Freak behavior: "I'm not a Germ Freak, but I never touch public restroom doorknobs." "I'm not a Germ Freak, but I bring my own sheets to hotels." Or the clincher, "I'm not a Germ Freak, but I wash my toothbrush with antibacterial soap before I brush my teeth." Ding, ding, ding: Germ Freak!

This is your call not to hide your head—or your HandiWipes. By outing ourselves, we can break the stereotypes that Germ Freaks are high maintenance or walking around in "haz mat" suits: Among us are professional athletes who don't flinch when a 250-pound opponent tries to tackle them, but who cower when someone sneezes near them (and rightly so); CEOs who value a cohesive team but excuse themselves from a meeting if someone is coughing; parents who expose their kids to more experiences than prior generations but not the pathogens that go with them. In a word (well, two) we are Germ Freaks. And we should be congratulated, not condoned; applauded, not made fun of (okay, you can make fun of us a little).

In this book I'll share the practical art of germ avoidance. You wouldn't step out in front of a car moving at fifty miles an hour, so why step in front of a sniffling person and be hit with a sneeze at ninety-three miles an hour? Most of us try to avoid inhaling other people's smoke, why not avoid inhaling their flu virus? I will show you how.

With the advice of infectious disease experts, you can stop wasting your time and money on things that supposedly guard against germs but may be totally useless—and downright harmful. You'll hear from other Germ Freaks: their pet peeves and guerilla tactics for staying healthy when everyone around them is hacking. You'll see what works, what's wasteful and what's just wacked.

In this age of time-crunched doctors, busy schedules and insurance companies that pay for less, it's in our own best interest to take control of our health. I hope to help us clean up our collective act when it comes to illness. To help sick people get a clue . . . or at least a tissue. If I can save you from even one cold or flu, this book has paid for itself—and at the very least, you can use it to secretly wipe your nose.

PART I

Germ Freak
Basics

Latent, Blatant or Wannabe: The Germ Freak Spectrum

It's okay to admit it: You're a Germ Freak. As with any other lifestyle that isn't mainstream, some people will misunderstand you, make fun of you or claim you're contributing to the downfall of society (i.e., "Your over-cleanliness is breeding mutant bugs"). The first step to owning your identity is acceptance.

Typically, Germ Freaks fall into four categories: latent, middle of the road, blatant or wannabes. Latent Germ Freaks hide their tendencies, perhaps letting down their guard when they're among friends or after a few drinks. Middle-of-the-road Germ Freaks are very levelheaded: They don't hoard instant hand sanitizer or remove their backyard bird feeder when the headlines scream "Avian Bird Flu"; they didn't put a moratorium on sugar during the anthrax scare because "You just never know." Blatant Germ Freaks don't hide their behavior; when someone calls them a Germ Freak, or the variants "nutcase" or "wacko," they take it as a compliment. And while there are very few Germ Freak wannabes at this point in time, look for the numbers to surge once more Germ Freaks come out of the closet and get the respect they deserve.

For the self-conscious Germ Freak, it might help to know that there are many famous Germ Freaks. It just takes a few celebrities to start a trend, like they did for the Atkins diet and Kabbalah. Instead of counting carbs, friends will swap secrets on reducing daily germ loads. Instead of Gap T-shirts on the red carpet, you'll see ones that say: HANDS OFF: PROPERTY OF A GERM FREAK. There are dating services for Jewish singles and adventurous singles; why not single Germ Freaks? At the very least you'd know you're having protected sex. But this will only be possible if Germ Freaks unite. So when you see another Germ Freak, give him or her a nod like runners do, a wave like Saturn owners or that "so you were up all night too?" look that mothers give when their strollers pass.

Famous Germ Freaks

NFL player **Randy Moss** won't touch doorknobs with his bare hands, frequently uses antibacterial soap and won't let anyone open his refrigerator without washing their hands. (*Blatant Germ Freak.*)

Comedian **Howie Mandel** built a guesthouse where he could stay when his kids get sick. (*Blatant. Maybe he just wanted to get some sleep.*)

P. Diddy reportedly wrote in a catering memo: "Before serving, all food and ice must be inspected for hair, package, paper, etc., and all catering staff must wear hairnets. Room must be stocked with twenty bars of Lever soap for showers (antibacterial) or Zest." (*Middle-of-the-road. Who likes hair in their food?*)

Cameron Diaz opens public doors with her elbows. (*Latent, and flexible too: Only 2 percent of Americans do this.*)

Donald Trump detests handshakes. "Shaking hands. It's a terrible custom. One of the worst. It's been proven you can get colds and flu and everything else. To me, the only good thing about shaking hands prior to eating is that I tend to eat less." (*Middle-of-the-road. Can you blame him? Think of how many hands he has to shake to close a deal.*)

Bianca Lawson, actress, Buffy the Vampire Slayer. "Usually [in an audition] it's a scene that involves a kiss, and this is when it gets weird. There are twenty girls in the waiting room, and all I can think is, *This guy has been kissing one girl after another, all day long.* You gotta do what you gotta do, but it's gross." (*Wannabe.*)

Drew Barrymore kissed her star on the Hollywood Walk of Fame as soon as it was unveiled on February 3, 2004, because she knew she couldn't kiss it after everybody had stood on it. She says, "I don't think I'm like a Howard Hughes germophobe or anything like that but I do think about that stuff." (*Latent . . . and possibly in denial.*)

The Quest for Immunity: Real-World *Survivor*

"Germs can help trigger our immune system, help
us digest food, help protect us from other, nastier
diseases, but don't kid yourself, germs are still
the number one killer on the planet."

PHILIP TIERNO, PH.D.
DIRECTOR OF CLINICAL MICROBIOLOGY AND IMMUNOLOGY
NEW YORK UNIVERSITY MEDICAL CENTER

Everyone knows we become prime targets for germs when
our immunity is low or when we're faced with an onslaught of
germs over an extended period of time. Really then, the cold and flu
season can be likened to a season of *Survivor*: A group of you start
out in an office—a corporate jungle filled with backstabbers, a bud-
ding couple and a few people who actually do some work. Days pass:

Some of you don't eat like you should; one of you doesn't get the sleep he needs and then loses immunity. After an intense meeting, *boom*, this unlucky guy finds himself back home, in bed, feeling awful and wondering when he can return to life as he knew it. And just like on the show, his untimely departure makes him the stuff of water-cooler conversation: "Poor guy . . ." "I didn't think he'd be the one who'd get it. . . ." "Do you think he'll be okay?"

Yes, in an ideal world we'd eat right, exercise and get at least seven hours of uninterrupted sleep a night. But does this always happen? *Ha!*

Evolution of Immune Compromisation
Parental Specimen

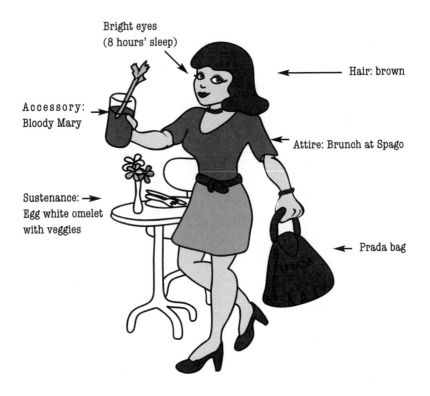

Bright eyes
(8 hours' sleep)

Hair: brown

Accessory:
Bloody Mary

Attire: Brunch at Spago

Sustenance: →
Egg white omelet
with veggies

Prada bag

1992 B.C. (Before Children)

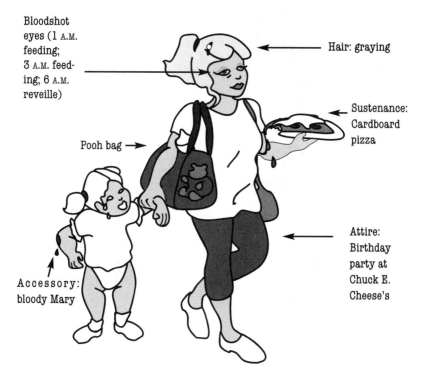

2005 A.D. (After Delivery)

Operation Germ Evasion

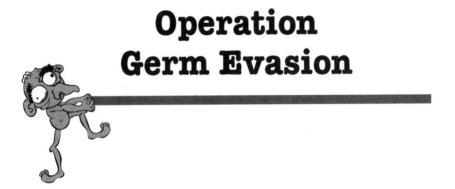

It doesn't matter what your B.C. is—Before Children, Before a Chronic Condition or Before a Career that leaves you jet-lagged and trapped on a plane with ten germ spreaders. If your immunity is down during cold and flu season, you'll likely be the next victim of whatever's going around. So without super immunity, you must be super vigilant.

If you want to survive, use all six germ avoidance techniques that follow.

Tactic #1: Avoid Germ Spreaders Like the Plague

When a person coughs or sneezes, they expel droplets that can travel 3 feet.

Avoiding germ spreaders isn't that hard. You already size people up when you scan a party for someone you know or scan a dark parking lot for a potential psycho (hopefully they're not the same person). Now you need to add to your radar people who look sick and be ready to avoid them. (See Field Guide to Germ Spreaders, page 12.) If you can't avoid them altogether, keep at least a three-foot distance from them and don't touch them. It just takes being cognizant and creative, as the following examples show.

Germ Spreader

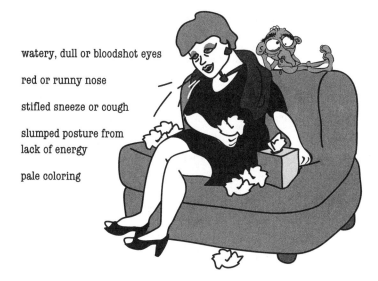

watery, dull or bloodshot eyes

red or runny nose

stifled sneeze or cough

slumped posture from lack of energy

pale coloring

Field Guide to Germ Spreaders

Male Species: The male species germ spreader displays an interesting dichotomy: When he experiences a life-threatening situation, like excruciating chest pains or a flesh-eating bacteria that's devouring his arm, he will say it was just the sausage he ate or poison ivy from mowing the lawn. However, when he feels the first sniffle or throat scratch of a minor cold, he will act as if he should be LifeFlighted to the best teaching hospital. Whenever the male genus is sick with a cold or flu, you will know it: They do everything loudly, act helpless and usually leave a trail of used, balled-up tissues.

Female Species: The female species is easier to spot in a sense than the male species because they are very in tune with their bodies, and like to take care of symptoms early with a therapeutic shopping trip. Their germ accoutrements may include echinacea tincture, a box of green tea, various Chinese herbs and a copy of Andrew Weil, M.D.'s *Optimal Healing*; if it's a very minor illness, the trip might include a new pair of shoes. However, because the female species has the benefit of eye concealer, foundation and lipstick, they often look quite healthy even when highly contagious.

Little Species: Most human specimens under five are either sick or about to be, so consider them perpetual germ spreaders.

Distinctive Sneezes: Look for the multiple sneeze, the stifled sneeze, the wet sneeze, the superwet sneeze, the wasabi-always-does-this-to-me sneeze (not necessarily contagious).

Distinctive Coughs: Listen for the hacking cough, the annoying cough, the seal cough, the goose cough, the-coughing-up-a-lung cough and the ah-hem cough.

Real-World Maneuver:
Dodging the Snotty Handshake

Is it firm enough? Does it feel like a wet noodle or that I'm trying too hard? You spent months early in your career nailing your handshake, and now that you've got it down you don't want to do it anymore. And there's a good reason: The handshake is a vector of viruses. So what can you do when you're finishing your presentation and hear "Achoo!"? And then another. And another. The meeting ends and The Sneezer extends his freshly coated hand. Your boss is watching to see if you can close the deal. What can you do?

Best Option: If you work at a granola-crunchy company, you can get away with a yoga bow or a forearm tap.

Good Option: Muster your best corporate voice and say: "Glad you're on the team. I'd shake your hand but I just had a serious sinus infection and don't want you to bring it home to your family." Make sure you get the words "serious" and "infection" in there, or you'll look like a big wimp.

Worst Option: If the client is very important and your boss is a real jerk, shake the person's hand and go immediately to the bathroom for a double hand wash up to your elbows.

Mark Cooper, the top elected official in Southbury, Connecticut, held a press conference to announce that he wouldn't shake any hands during the flu season of 2004 to 2005. Instead of offering his hand, he offered people a pamphlet titled, "Don't Do the Flu." He explains, "I go to a holiday event and shake 300 hands. Those people are picking up food and they are shaking hands with each other. If you come into contact with someone like me in that context, you might want to think twice about shaking my hand."

During the same flu season, the Roman Catholic Diocese of Metuchen, New Jersey, told parishioners that they could smile, bow or wave instead of shaking hands during the Sign of Peace. Vermont Bishop Kenneth Angell urged Catholic churches to abstain from shaking hands from Christmas to Easter prompting priests to hold "flu-free gatherings."

Real-World Maneuver:
Evading the Sneezer in the Elevator

Always practice Elevator Surveillance before you get in because once the doors close, you're trapped. If anyone looks the least bit sick, don't get in. If you're in a group, fake an urgent voice: "Oops, I forgot my cell phone." **Note:** This won't work if you're holding your phone in your hand. If you're with a fellow Germ Freak, call the sick person's

bluff and say very loudly: "So, you haven't started taking the antibiotics for that bacterial thingie yet?" You need to say this convincingly
enough so that the sick person exits immediately. This rarely works
because there's not enough time to say it. If you get trapped in an elevator and hear someone sniffle, push the button to get off on the next
floor—even if it's not yours—and hold your breath until you get out.
Walk to your destination; it's better for you anyway.

Tactic #2:
Don't Touch Germ Hot Spots

 The SARS (Severe Acute Respiratory Syndrome) virus
can survive on plastic surfaces, such as elevator buttons, for up to 24 hours.

While the headlines scream of mad cow disease, Ebola and flesh-
eating bacteria, you are far more likely to be knocked off your feet
by the cold you catch from your office desk. While most of us
wouldn't purposely go out and jump headfirst into a vat of Ebola,
each day we unknowingly do the equivalent: When you touch the
shopping cart handle laden with E. coli and then sample the deli
turkey, your life could literally be in your own hands. Throughout
the book Danger Zone icons 🔴 will alert you to the most contaminated spots you likely touch (or not) each day. Disinfect these
areas and/or follow proper hand-washing procedures (see page 21)
after touching them.

Real-World Maneuver:
Jockeying Around Public Bathroom Doorknobs

Listen up, Germ Freaks: Public bathroom doorknobs are definitely a germ hot spot but not quite like you think. The *outside* doorknob is actually germier than the inside knob. For Germ Freaks who fear the knob, use the following strategies:

Perfect-World Option: Time your departure with someone else's arrival and skate out without making contact with the doorknob. This is not a recommended if you are in a low-traffic area.

Best Option: Use a tissue to cover the handle or knob and then throw it in the trash. If there's no trashcan, throw the tissue on the floor and eventually management will get a clue. Don't feel bad— experts actually recommend this method.

Good Option: Use your opposite hand (left hand if you're right-handed) to open the door and wash it as soon as you can. Chances are you're less likely to touch your nose, mouth or eyes with your nondominant hand.

Decent Option: Grab the handle with your pinky (or index finger) so that you have only a one in ten chance of touching anything important if you forget to wash later. You never use your pinky anyway.

Pushing-It Option: Open the door using your sleeve as a covering. Just remember to wash your shirt when you get home.

Desperation: Say you're in the bathroom with someone and you don't want them to think you're, well, a freak who can't touch a doorknob . . . what to do? Eyeball the handle and go for the part you think has been touched the least.

A Germ Freak's ✓GOTTA HAVE IT?

With the slogan, "When in doubt, whip it out," who wouldn't want a **Wakmah,** a multipurpose plastic sucker that fits in your pocket? You can mount the Wakmah on any surface, and the powerful suction cup will open a germy bathroom door, stand-in as a hook to hold your purse in a public bathroom, or become your personal handle on a crowded subway (for even more uses go to: *www.i-suck.com*). Contact: *www.Wakmah.co.uk.* For inquiring minds, Wakmah is short for Watercloset Aperture Kinetic Mechanical Activation Handle (plus it was free as a domain name) . . . and, yes, it was invented in the UK.

Germs on the Subway

"If someone is coughing on the subway,
I get off at the next stop. I'd rather walk and
be late for work than get loogied on."

A FREQUENTLY TARDY GERM FREAK

So you think the subway is a germy cesspool? Well, you're mostly right. In 2003, the *New York Daily News* took swab samples from 49 locations across New York's mass transit system. Here's a sample of what they found: A subway station escalator handrail had strep B, *Streptococcus viridans*, E. coli, enterococcus; a subway platform had *Aspergillus*, penicillium molds; a subway ticket machine had strep A, E. coli, enterococcus; and subway trains had *Streptococcus viridans*, enterococcus and E. coli.

 Have your coffee and bagel when you reach your destination, not on the subway.

Real-World Maneuver: Just Saying No to Community Foodstuffs

 When a person has a cold, they are most likely to transmit it to you on the second to fourth day of infection, when the nasal secretions are the highest.

It seems like every week you're trying to dig up spare change and pen a pithy message for an office birthday card. While it's bad enough to be the birthday honoree who has to feign surprise when you walk in to a dark cafeteria full of twenty coworkers yelling "Shhh" at the top of their lungs, it's excruciating to be a Germ Freak attendee: We know that when the candles are blown out with an exhale of virus, we'll be expected to partake in infectious disease.

During cold and flu season, avoid community food celebrations altogether—except, of course, when it's your boss's birthday, when you should go for the singing only. If you need an excuse, tell everyone you're on a diet (germ-free, that is). People tend to think Germ Freaks are, well, freaks, but they think you're noble if you're avoiding excess calories instead of deadly pathogens.

Always beware of the tower of bagels: Someone did a lot of groping to get them into this formation. The rest of the people had to touch at least one or two bagels to get to the one they wanted. If a bagel fell—which it most likely did, given the law of gravity—they tried to reposition it and sighed (big germy exhale) when they couldn't.

Never eat the raisin bagels. These are almost always picked up many times over and then discarded when people realize they contain raisins, not chocolate bits. Don't sneak a bagel hours after the soiree, unless you'd like some salmonella with your cream cheese.

 TIP Avoid holiday food baskets, especially the homemade ones where the end result looks like a small child assisted the chef.

Germs on the Dating Scene

"My ex-boyfriend used to get really sick
every year and be coughing up different colors.
Since we shared a house and a mortgage I had no
option but to sleep on the couch all the time.
Today, if I'm dating anyone who coughs more
than a 'change of season adjustment cough,' I
dump him. I'd rather be healthy than a couple."

A VERY SINGLE GERM FREAK

Don't think you need to spend your life alone. Germ Freaks can
still date; they just need to think of some creative alternatives to
some worst-case dating scenarios:

Bowling: How many people have put their sweaty feet in those
shoes? And how many people have palmed the balls? **Germ
Freak Alternative:** Rollerblading in the open air.

Asian Food: Dim sum = don't have some! Raw sushi? A community
bowl of edamame beans? **Germ Freak Alternative:** Italian food;
it's hard to split a plate of spaghetti.

Movies: Sharing a bucket of popcorn in a crowded theater. **Germ
Freak Alternative:** Offbeat less-crowded matinee; no need to get
popcorn because you'll be eating dinner after.

Speed Dating: A fast track to germs, not the altar. **Germ Freak
Alternative:** *Match.com.* A great way to meet people without
contaminating yourself . . . until later.

Studies have shown fecal germs on movie theater head-rests and Candida on the seats.

Tactic #3: Wash Your Hands Correctly (Only 16% of Us Do)

"We watched people in movie theaters:
Only 67% of them even washed their hands; only
half of those people used soap;
only half of those washed their hands for
the 20 seconds needed, so really only
16% of people came out with their
hands washed adequately."

DR. GERBA

Despite what you might think, hot water isn't necessary to remove germs from your hands. Washing with warm water is best because if the water is too hot or cold, people tend to stop washing before the germs are lifted. Use plain, old-fashioned hand soap and save the souped-up soaps for special situations (see page 34).

Hand Washing 101

Wet your hands and lather the soap all over, rubbing between your fingers, the top and palm of your hands and under your nails. It's this friction that gets the germs off, so rub for a full fifteen seconds (don't do this under the faucet or you'll wash the soap off too soon). Rinse your hands thoroughly. The whole process should take at least twenty seconds. Some people sing "Yankee Doodle Dandy" or "Happy Birthday" to get to their allotted twenty seconds; the silent renditions are recommended. Some parents teach their kids to sing the ABC song; this only works if your children don't get stuck at the letter F.

Wash your hands frequently throughout the day, and at least at these key times:

- Before you eat
- After you use the bathroom
- After you touch an animal
- After you come in from the outside
- After you cough or sneeze (this is to protect others from your germs)
- After touching raw meat, fish or poultry while cooking
- After you change a diaper or a tampon
- When they're visibly dirty (Duh.)

Tactic #4: Stop Touching Your Face (You Just Did It Again)

 The average person touches her mouth, nose, eyes and ears one to three times every five minutes. The average child does this ten times every five minutes.

Don't touch your face or ears until you wash your hands. Stop doing this! You just did it again. Really, you've got to find a new nervous habit.

Tactic #5: Wipe Germs Out, Don't Just Wipe Them Around

The common cold virus can survive up to three days outside the nasal passages on objects and surfaces. 70% of people who have a cold have infectious germs on their hands.

When zapping germs with a disinfectant or sanitizer, your goal is to reduce their numbers to a safe level rather than eliminate them completely. While most of us detest reading directions, you should, because too many people use disinfecting products and wipe them off after a few seconds. "The worst thing you could do is to use these products very diluted and very occasionally. If you give bacteria a chance, they will mutate," explains Kansas University professor Lester Mitscher, a medical chemist who has worked in antibiotic research since the 1950s. So unless you want your kids toting mutant bugs to their science fair, follow the directions. The main thing to remember is you have to kill these guys, not move them around.

Disinfecting 101

When using a commercial cleaning product, make sure the label says "disinfecting" or "sanitizing," or else you can't guarantee the product will be effective. When you sanitize something, you go a step beyond cleaning; when you disinfect it, you go a step beyond sanitizing. While some people mix their own environmentally friendly products, the only way to guarantee you're killing certain germs is to buy a commercial cleaner with a container label or product fact sheet that has an EPA (Environmental Protection Agency) number. All commercial disinfectants register their effectiveness claims with the EPA, so if the product label claims to kill *Staphylococcus aureus,* test data must be submitted to prove it. Without the EPA number, you can't be sure.

Stuart Levy, physician and microbiologist at Tufts University School of Medicine, recommends a return to tried-and-true cleansers like alcohol, chlorine bleach and hydrogen peroxide that leave no residues like antibacterial cleaners do. If you want to go this route, the Centers for Disease Control and Prevention (CDC) recommends using a mixture of one gallon of warm water to three-quarters a cup of bleach. You'll need to clean the surface area of dirt and grime, and let the bleach solution sit for ten minutes before rinsing.

Whenever you disinfect, wear gloves (and a mask if you're sensitive to chemicals), open windows, turn on ceiling fans, and send the kids out to play or in a room away from the chemicals.

Down-and-Dirty Cleaning When Someone in the House Is Sick

 Introduction of the flu virus into a household by one family member usually causes disease in two-thirds of other family members.

In many households, the start of school followed by flu season begins a revolving door of respiratory and other ills. By using the following tactics when the first sniffle erupts, you can make sure your whole family doesn't go along for the ride.

- Disinfect the following items whenever the sick person touches them (if you're not sure, disinfect them anyway):

light switches	sink faucet handles
phones	shared games and toys
remote control	pretty much everything in
microwave handle	the bathroom (sink/counter/
refrigerator handle	faucet/doorknob/toilet handle)
kitchen counters	

- Use paper towels (made from recycled materials) in the bathroom and kitchen instead of hand towels and dishcloths for the duration of the illness.

- Move all toothbrushes away from the sick person's (if you have more than one bathroom, use it until the person is better). Disinfect all toothbrushes with Listerine and dry them completely. Buy everyone a new toothbrush once the person is better.

- Buy each member of the household their own toothpaste (most people touch the toothpaste against the brush when dispensing).
- Wash all towels and facecloths after every use.
- If you share a bed with the sick person, sleep with the window open (or move to the couch).
- Wash the sick person's sheets and pillowcase every day.
- Keep all the windows in the house open if weather permits.
- If the sick person is a toddler, wash stuffed animals and favorite blankets in the washing machine; disinfect toys.

Tactic #6: Practice Proper Respiratory Etiquette

When you sneeze, air and particles leave your mouth and nose at 93 miles per hour.

I was recently at a restaurant, holding my two-year-old daughter up to see a fish tank. As she was watching the fish, an elderly man exited the restroom behind us, blasting out a coughing-up-a-lung cough right in my daughter's face. Was he totally clueless or had he lost all control of his bodily functions?

I yelled after him: "Thank you for sharing your disease with my daughter." My husband cringed (*Oh, no, not again*). The man turned around.

I followed with, "Sir, do you realize you just coughed on my daughter?" (It's important to begin any Germ Freak ranting with "Sir" or "Ma'am.") He looked dumbfounded.

"Oh, sorry." He walked away.

While it's doubtful my words had any effect on him, they needed to be said. We shouldn't feel too nice to tell oblivious people they're violating Respiratory Etiquette when they assault us with their germs. Forget obnoxious Public Displays of Affection; Public Displays of Infection must be viewed as more than a social faux pas.

In Port Arthur, Texas, it's against the law to emit "obnoxious odors" in an elevator. But flatulence won't kill you, although some may beg to differ. In Alaska, public flatulence carries a $100 fine; why not fine public coughing without covering your mouth?

The good news for Germ Freaks, and for the world at large, is people are starting to talk about respiratory etiquette. Copy the following page and tape it onto your refrigerator at home or work, or put it on someone's car dashboard if you don't want to confront a germ spreader directly:

Respiratory Etiquette Manifesto: Learn It, Live It, Pass It On

Eight Ways to Keep Your Germs from Spreading

· Cover your mouth or nose with a tissue when you sneeze or cough and throw the tissue away (no germy handkerchiefs!).

· If you don't have a tissue, cough or sneeze into your elbow sleeve, *not your hand*.

· Wash your hands often with regular hand soap and water and always after you sneeze or cough.

· Use an alcohol-based hand sanitizer when you can't wash with regular soap and water.

· If you're sick, stay home. If you can't stay home, don't go near children, pregnant women or anyone who is immune compromised.

· If you're sick, don't fly.

· If you go to a hospital with a high fever or rash, let people know: They may want to give you a mask.

· Realize that you may be contagious two days before you're sick and up to a week after.

If You Must Be in Public When Sick

· Rethink your decision: Are you really that important? Couldn't you use a little downtime?

Real-World Maneuver: Making Party Conversation with Non-Germ Freaks

If you haven't already encountered the following comments from non–Germ Freaks, you will soon. So you won't be caught off guard, here are some answers. Memorize them and they'll fly off your tongue at the next dinner party.

Non–Germ Freak Comment: "Don't avoid getting sick because being sick gives your immune system a workout."

Answer: Option 1: "You're an idiot." Option 2: "Are you volunteering to come to my house when my four-year-old triplets are getting a chicken pox power workout?" Option 3: "I'll remember that comment the next time you call me complaining you have the flu."

Non–Germ Freak Comment: "I read about this hygiene hypothesis that says being too clean is causing increased illness."

Answer: Option 1: "I didn't think you knew how to read." Option 2: "Using soap properly has never killed anyone, but not using soap has. If you don't appreciate the luxury of soap, take your next vacation to a third-world country—you'll realize just how fortunate you are."

Non–Germ Freak Comment: "Children who grow up in homes that are too clean are more likely to have asthma."

Germ Freak Answer: Option 1: "Do you really think a home that has kids in it can *ever* be too clean?" Option 2: "Then your kids are safe because your house is a real dump." Option 3: "Not true. Dust mites are linked to 50 to 80 percent of U.S. asthma cases and cockroaches are a major asthma trigger. You don't find cockroaches and dust bunnies in superclean homes."

Non–Germ Freak Comment: "Back in my day, we mothers never worried about germs and our babies didn't get sick."

Germ Freak Answer: Option 1: "Back in your day you also thought it was okay to pile five kids in the back of a station wagon without seatbelts. Thank goodness for progress." Option 2: "Back in your day, most mothers stayed home and kids played with siblings. Today's kids start some type of 'school' before they're two, where they'll lay on a mat, pick up Play-Doh or mouth a rattle that fifty other kids have drooled on that morning."

Germ Freak Essentials

Vigilance is one thing; product readiness is another. Here's a list of essentials that no Germ Freak should be without. A word of advice: go forth and gather supplies before you need them. Like bees to honey go sick people to the medicine aisle, so you don't want to linger here during cold and flu season comparing prices or sorting coupons. Know what you need, then grab and go.

Germ Freaks on the Go:
Purses and Briefcases

❏ To-go pack of toilet paper (*www.cottonbuds.com*)
❏ To-go pack of toilet seat covers (*www.cottonbuds.com*
   or *www.cleansleeve.com*)
❏ Travel-size instant hand sanitizer (to be used when soap
   and water is unavailable)
❏ Disinfecting wipes or rubbing alcohol pads
❏ Band-Aids (not antibacterial)
❏ Tissues

At Home

❏ Pump dispenser soap (not antibacterial)
❏ Disinfectant cleaner or sanitizer
❏ Recyclable paper towels
❏ Tissues
❏ Listerine or hydrogen peroxide (to disinfect toothbrushes)
❏ Rubber gloves (think disinfecting, not daywear)
❏ Bleach

Supplements

❏ **Airborne.** This effervescent formula was created by a
   teacher who was sick of getting sick. A combination of seven
   herbal extracts, antioxidants, electrolytes and vitamin C,
   you take it before going into crowded areas (like planes) or
   at the first sign of a cold. Both celebrities and everyday
   Germ Freaks swear by it. *www.airbornehealth.com.*

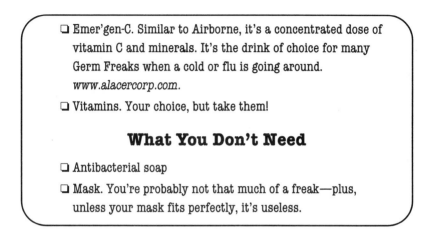

❏ Emer'gen-C. Similar to Airborne, it's a concentrated dose of vitamin C and minerals. It's the drink of choice for many Germ Freaks when a cold or flu is going around. *www.alacercorp.com.*

❏ Vitamins. Your choice, but take them!

What You Don't Need

❏ Antibacterial soap

❏ Mask. You're probably not that much of a freak—plus, unless your mask fits perfectly, it's useless.

The Dirt on Antibacterial Soap

In 2004, Americans purchased more than $540 million worth of antibacterial soaps, hand cleaners and detergents. Seventy-five percent of liquid and 29 percent of bar soaps on the market are antibacterial. What does this mean, other than that we are a nation of Germ Freaks? It means a lot of us are wasting our money.

A March 2004 study in the *Annals of Internal Medicine* showed that people who use antibacterial soaps instead of regular hand soap had the same number of colds, runny noses, sore throats and fevers as those who used regular soap. Antibacterial soaps don't prevent colds or flu because they are caused by viruses, not bacteria.

Even Worse . . .

Some manufacturers list their product as antibacterial when the antibacterial agent, usually triclosan, is only used as a preservative or in very small quantities. Therefore, many of the antibacterial soaps you're paying for don't have enough oomph to fully kill germs. Since soap manufacturers aren't required to list the antibacterial concentration of their products, there's no way to know if the soap you're buying even works against a hardier bacteria unless you call their 800 number and ask. (How many hours do you think you'll be on hold to ask this one?) Plus, unless you're a microbiologist, you have no way of knowing if the germs in your sink need a small dose or a big one, or if they're bacterial or viral. There have even been lab studies that show triclosan breaks down human skin cells. Why pay extra money for a soap that might hurt you?

According to Nancy Tomes, history professor at the State University of New York at Stony Brook, antibacterial soaps were designed to capitalize on the general public's emerging germ fears to sell more soap, not to fight germs. "If you have HIV [or another disease], then you need to be more careful than the rest of us," Tomes explained. "But the advertising on television isn't aimed at the sick. It's aimed at the normal." So, if you're a "normal" American (or just pretending to be), forgo the antibacterial soap.

When to Use Antibacterial Soap

· If you're working in a medical setting.
· If you're immune compromised (ask your doctor).

Antibacterial Products:
A Little Dab Will Do Ya . . . In?

What if you're visiting a friend and the soap in her bathroom is antibacterial: Will you be breeding antibacterial-resistant germs if you use it? Relax, using antibacterial products *in small amounts* won't cause superbugs. However, if the soap in your workplace bathroom is antibacterial, and you wash your hands many times a day, you'd be better off bringing your own plain hand soap. While none of the theories about mutant bugs have been proven in the real world, why take a chance?

Eugene Cole, professor at Brigham Young University in Salt Lake City, Utah, conducted studies to determine whether people who used antibacterial products regularly would cause antibacterial resistance. In a randomized study of thirty homes that used antibacterial products and thirty that did not, they took bacterial samples from occupants' heads and mouths and surroundings. The research showed that antibiotic resistance was *not* an issue in homes where antibacterial products were used. The Food and Drug Administration had an independent panel of medical experts in 1997 review the available data on bacterial resistance due to antibacterial wash products. The conclusion: no link between the use of the products and bacterial resistance.

Use Them Judiciously and Correctly

However, Stuart Levy, a Tufts University School of Medicine physician and microbiologist cautions, "Dousing everything we

touch with antibacterial soaps and taking antibiotic medications at
the first sign of a cold can upset the natural balance of microorganisms in and around us, leaving behind only the 'superbugs.' By
encouraging this 'unnatural selection' of bacteria that have grown
immune to most if not all of today's antibiotics, we unwittingly
endanger global health."

Squashing Superbugs

If your dab of antibacterial soap isn't causing antibacterial resistance, then what is? Most likely, America's overuse of antibiotics.
Doctors write 50 million unnecessary antibiotic prescriptions every
year, according to the Centers for Disease Control and Prevention.
Of those, 18 million are for the common cold and 6 million for sore
throats.

The meat and poultry most of us eat every day are pumped full
of antibiotics to improve their health and speed their development.
We get up in arms if an athlete takes steroids, yet we eat steak on
steroids without a thought. If you want to do your part to battle
antibacterial resistance, do the following:

- If you have a cold or the flu, hit your pillow before hitting up
  your doctor for antibiotics.
- If your doctor prescribes an antibiotic, ask why. (Antibiotics
  treat bacterial infections only; ask if the antibiotic prescribed
  specifically targets the source of your infection, and ensure that
  it's the narrowest spectrum drug possible.)

- Follow the dosing directions; don't stop the antibiotic even if you feel better.
- They're antibiotics, not Altoids: No sharing.
- If your child has chronic ear infections that require antibiotics (many do not), research using eardrops or homeopathic methods.
- Buy organic foods from manufacturers that don't feed their animals antibiotics. Investigate buying kosher foods.
- After taking a course of antibiotics, ask your doctor about taking probiotics to help reestablish healthy bacteria in your system.

GERM FREAK LEAST WANTED: ORTHOMYXOVIRUS

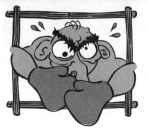

Street Name: The Flu.

Style: The Strong-Armed Bully. He preys on the elderly, children and anyone weaker than he is.

Modus Operandi: A one-two punch that knocks you off your feet; in some cases he won't stop until major damage is done.

Symptoms: Extreme fatigue; body aches; chills; headache; fever.

Contagiousness: Adults: one day before falling ill and three to seven days after symptoms develop; children may be contagious longer than a week.

Mode of Transmission: Respiratory secretions.

If You See This Germ: Know what you're dealing with. The three main types of influenza are A, B and C. Influenza C causes only mild disease while influenza types A and B cause dangerous epidemics nearly every year. During flu season, usually one or more influenza A subtype and B viruses circulate at the same time. Each year, in April, members of the World Health Organization announce their recommendation for the vaccines to be used in the upcoming flu season based on tracking information.

To track this germ nationwide, go to: *www.cdc.gov/flu/weekly/*.

Panic or Pandemic?

A pandemic is possible when an influenza A virus makes a dramatic change or shift. This shift results in a new virus to which the general population has no immunity. In order for a pandemic to occur, this novel virus must spread easily from person to person and must jump to more than one continent. So don't panic (yet!), but be prepared.

To Get the Vaccine or Not to Get the Vaccine . . . That Is the Question

Don't talk politics, religion or whether or not to get a flu shot around mixed company: Talk to your doctor instead. Also check out the CDC Web site for flu information. If you decide to get a shot, do it early in the season. And one thing's for certain: If you're waiting in a crowded VFW hall or supermarket to get a shot, you're exposing yourself to a megadose of germs. Schedule an appointment with your personal physician rather than waiting shoulder-to-shoulder with a hundred other people.

GERM FREAK LEAST WANTED: NOROVIRUS

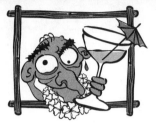

Street Name: Norwalk Virus, aka the stomach flu.

Style: The Social Butterfly. His charm is so contagious that you almost can't help but catch what he's got.

Modus Operandi: Flits from person to person on cruise ships, in day care centers, schools and offices, leaving a memorable calling card. Norovirus can live in an uncleaned carpet for a month.

Symptoms: Diarrhea, vomiting (the projectile type), stomach cramps that can last 12 to 60 hours.

Mode of Transmission: Person-to-person contact with infected person; improper food handling; touching a contaminated surface or food and then touching your mouth.

Incubation Period: Symptoms begin 24 to 48 hours after contact with virus.

If You See This Germ: Remember that he is highly contagious: The infectious dose is believed to be very small, less than 100 particles, although some think that as few as ten particles may produce disease.

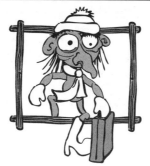

Street Name: The Common Cold.

Style: The Annoying Houseguest. She descends upon you in the wintertime and stays five days when you thought you'd be rid of her in two. And guess what? She'll be back again in three weeks.

Modus Operandi: She wears you down.

Symptoms: Runny nose, sore throat, cough, congestion, swollen glands, muscle aches and possible fever.

Mode of Transmission: Respiratory secretions or droplets when a person sneezes or coughs; hand-to-hand contact.

Incubation Period: Symptoms appear one to three days after contact with the virus.

If You See This Germ: Don't believe the rumors. You won't catch a cold from being outside or being wet unless an infected person coughs or sneezes on you. You don't need to see a doctor about a cold unless you have underlying medical problems, your cold has lasted more than two weeks or you notice new, bothersome symptoms including very thick, deeply colored mucus, facial pain and persistent fever. Viral infections, like colds, do *not* improve with antibiotics. If you have a question, call your doctor.

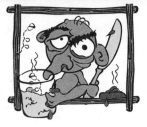

Street Name: E. coli

Style: The Backstabber

Modus Operandi: E. coli is usually a friend who helps us fight off predatory bacteria in our bodies; however, E. coli 0157:H7 can turn nasty, causing hemolytic uremic syndrome (HUS), a serious disease that affects children in particular. While most people with HUS recover after a prolonged hospital stay, it can cause fatal kidney failure.

Method of Transmission: Eating food or water containing the bacteria; person-to-person transmission if infected people don't wash their hands after using the toilet; contact with animal fecal microbes at zoos or petting zoos; improperly disinfected swimming pools.

Symptoms: Diarrhea, which may or may not be bloody; very bad abdominal cramps; possible fever or possible vomiting.

Incubation Period: Symptoms usually appear about three days after exposure, with a range of one to nine days.

If You See This Germ: Be aggressive. The symptoms of this infection are similar to other foodborne illnesses, so don't accept a diagnosis of "stomach virus" without insisting on a complete evaluation.

S.T.O.P.

The organization Safe Tables Our Priority (S.T.O.P.), recommends that at the first visit to the doctor, regardless of how bloody the stool is, parents should insist that the lab run separate tests for each of these: 1) shigella; 2) campylobacter; 3) salmonella; 4) shiga toxin or veotoxin test (indicates an E. coli infection) and 5) a MacConkey-sorbitol test for E. coli O157:H7. Meridian Diagnostics offers a faster test than the MacConkey-sorbitol test, but many doctors are unaware it exists (Meridian Diagnostics: 513-271-3700). If a physician recommends antibiotics or drugs like Kaopectate, ask why: Studies show antibiotics can severely worsen the infection. If your child develops HUS, insist that he or she be transferred to the best children's hospital. For more information, go to *www.safetables.org*.

As many as 15% of children who are infected with E. coli O157:H7 develop HUS. Approximately 7,500 cases of hemolytic uremic syndrome are diagnosed each year in the U.S., similar to the rate of incidence for leukemia in the general population.

Do You Need an Intervention?
When Your Habits Get Out of Control

Okay, so you've outfitted your cold and flu essentials, you know how to identify a germ spreader from three feet away and you know some infectious diseases to look out for. Now that your Germ Freak habits are becoming more ingrained, be careful you don't go overboard. Take this quiz to see if you may be going a bit too far, checking off any that apply:

❏ Your disinfecting is interfering with your ability to work. (Hmm, I think I'll just give the photocopier one more wipe . . . okay, maybe two.)

❏ Your habits are affecting your marriage. (Your spouse suspects you are downloading Internet porn or Googling ex-boyfriends, but you're really spending hours online tracking flu activity and looking up suspicious symptoms on WebMD.)

❏ You think about germs when you're alone. (Just how many millions of dust mites are on this pillow?)

❏ Other people have commented on your disinfecting. ("No, I don't need a HandiWipe. What's your problem?")

❏ You try to hide your germ habit. (Maybe he won't notice if I grab the bathroom door handle with my sleeve.)

❏ Your disinfecting is affecting your physical health. (You have red chafing on your hands from too much instant hand sanitizer.)

If you didn't check any boxes, you are a levelheaded middle-of-the-road Germ Freak.

If you checked two boxes, keep an eye on your habits.

If you checked three or more, you're over the top. Seek help immediately . . . or at least after the flu season ends.

PART II

The Daily Grime

The Home Front

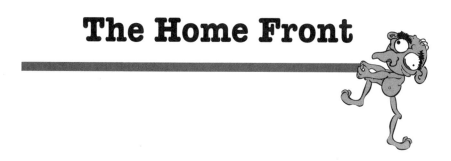

"I once thought the toughest job in the world was being the parent of a Little League pitcher. Now I know better. It's being the only healthy person in a house full of sick people."

RALPH DE LA CRUZ, REPORTER, *THE SUN-SENTINEL*

The stack of mail overtaking your kitchen counter, the laundry pile waiting to be folded, the shoe that doesn't have a match . . . all of these are telltale signs that you can be a Germ Freak without being a neat freak. While I envy people who have immaculate houses, I comfort my domestically challenged self with the fact that even if a house *looks* sparkly clean or clutter-free, it could be hiding germs. You don't have to be an obsessive cleaner to stay healthy (unless you want to be), but you do have to know where the germs are hanging out in your home.

The Germiest Things in Your Home

- Kitchen dishcloth
- Kitchen sink
- Toilet bowl
- Kitchen garbage can
- Refrigerator
- Bathroom doorknob
- Cutting board

Kitchen

"Your kitchen harbors more germs than any other room in the home. The greatest germ concentration is found in the kitchen sponges and dishcloths. Sink drains, faucet handles, and door-knobs—either in the kitchen or bathroom—were the next highest on the list."

The Journal of Applied Microbiology

Sponges and Dishcloths

Don't use the sponge or dishcloth from the kitchen to "clean" the dining room table. Disinfect the sponge or dishcloth every time you use it to wipe up meat or vegetables and then let it dry. The best and easiest way to make sure a nonabrasive, cellulose sponge is safe is to put it in the microwave for two minutes while it's damp. (Don't burn your hands when you take it out.) You can also run it through the dishwasher. Replace your sponges biweekly; use paper towels made from recycled materials instead of sponges during flu season.

 The average kitchen sponge can harbor 7.2 billion germs.

The Sink

"If an alien came from space and studied bacterial counts in the typical home, he would probably conclude he should wash his hands in your toilet and pee in your sink."

Dr. Gerba

Disinfect your sink weekly, especially the faucet handle; during flu season, or if someone is contagious, disinfect it daily.

 90% of kitchen sinks carry salmonella.

Fridge

Buy a refrigerator thermometer to ensure that your fridge is between 34° and 40° Fahrenheit. If something spills in your fridge, wipe it up immediately. Give your fridge a thorough cleaning every three months.

If you're having a party and will be opening and closing the refrigerator door frequently, turn down the temperature a few degrees.

Refrigerate leftovers promptly. Bacteria can grow quickly at room temperature, so refrigerate leftover foods within ninety minutes. Large volumes of food will cool more quickly if they are divided into several shallow containers for refrigeration.

Counters

DANGER ZONE Wash counters with hot soapy water after meal prep; disinfect them if raw meat trouched them. Sanitize them daily or if someone in the house is sick.

Cutting Boards

"If you have a choice between licking a cutting board or a toilet seat . . . pick the toilet seat."

Dr. Gerba

DANGER ZONE Buy two different cutting boards—one for meat and one for vegetables and fruit. Put the cutting board in the dishwasher after you use it; don't just give it a quick rinse. While different theories abound whether plastic or wood cutting boards are best to reduce germs, the safest way to ensure you kill any germs is to give them a thorough washing no matter what kind you buy. Don't use a homemade bleach solution to clean wooden cutting boards because the wood neutralizes the disinfectant properties of the bleach.

Use Them or Lose Them?
Antibacterial Cutting Boards

Lose them. Earth to consumer: *Helloooo*. You buy an antibacterial cutting board and then put raw chicken on it . . . you just contaminated it. You buy an antibacterial teething toy and your baby drools on it . . . you just contaminated it. You still need to use basic cleaning and care. Buying antibacterial products may give some people a false sense of security. Better to save your money and stock up on regular soap.

Garbage

Disinfect the garbage can once a week.

Kitchen Floor

Wipe up spills as soon as they happen; disinfect the floor weekly, more if you have toddlers who eat food they drop. Don't encourage the "five-second rule" in your house because food can become contaminated within five seconds in the right conditions.

Garbage Disposal

Always cover the garbage disposal while running it because droplets of spray can get on your counters or food. Don't let food build up in the disposal. Run it every time you put something down it and let the water run for fifteen to twenty seconds after you are done to rinse the by-products away. Disinfect the disposal weekly.

Dining In

"Most people associate foodborne illness with improperly cooked foods of animal origin, but the fact is, the number of people getting sick from eating fruits and vegetables contaminated with pathogens has doubled [to 76 million a year] since 1990."

Ann Draughon, Codirector, University of Tennessee Food Safety Center of Excellence

"50% to 80% of all foodborne illnesses originate in the home. Tell this to your spouse the next time you need an excuse to go out to eat."

Dr. Gerba

While vegetables and fruits cause an estimated 20 to 25 percent of annual food illness cases, meat, poultry, pork and eggs still cause about 40 to 45 percent of illnesses. Seafood and cheeses also account for a large percentage of foodborne illness. To minimize the risk, take these precautions:

Produce

Wash all produce for at least thirty seconds using the sprayer. Scrub produce that has skin with a produce brush or peel off the skin. (A produce brush is the best option because the fiber is in the skin.)

Lettuce

Remove the outer leaves of lettuce or cabbage. Wash each leaf under running water. Don't submerge the entire head in water or you'll just be rinsing it in contaminated water. Even though some of the prepackaged salad mixes and cut-up veggies say "prewashed," don't believe it. Wash them again.

Use Them or Lose Them? Produce Sprays

Lose them. The sprays that are sold to clean pesticides off of produce sometimes contain other chemicals. And while they may effectively remove pesticides, they don't remove all microorganisms or the sneeze from the guy in aisle three. By washing all produce thoroughly and by scrubbing fruits with skin, you will remove the pesticides—with the germs. If you're concerned about pesticides, save your money on the sprays and buy organic foods.

Cantaloupe

Three multistate outbreaks of salmonella have been associated with eating cantaloupe imported from Mexico. Always scrub the outside of the cantaloupe and wash the fruit well *after* you cut it. The reason? The knife goes through the rind and takes any dirt (or other items) on the outside to the inside.

Alfalfa Sprouts

The poor alfalfa sprout. First it had a reputation as a hippie food, and now it's being implicated as a source of salmonella. Sprouts are grown in warm, moist conditions—the perfect environment for bacteria. Unfortunately, the contamination occurs in the seed itself, so it's very difficult to remove the bacteria. If you have a healthy immune system, eat sprouts with caution; if you are immune compromised, don't eat them.

Chicken

Many health-conscious people have replaced the red meat they used to eat for chicken. Unfortunately, commercial chickens are dirty birds. It's best to purchase organic, grass-fed poultry whenever possible. Rinse chicken well and cook it thoroughly. If someone complains it's dry, tell them, "Better dry than to die."

More than 50% of chickens sold in grocery stores carry bacteria that can make people sick if they are not cooked thoroughly.

Ground Meat or Turkey

"The more you handle something, the greater chance that bacteria is introduced," says Lisa Lachenmayr, extension educator in nutrition and food safety with the University of Maryland Cooperative Extension Service. "[When] it's ground, it goes through more machines and has a greater chance of introducing bacteria to the product." In other words, cook all meat thoroughly, especially burgers.

Some Like It Hot

To test the temperature of meat, poultry and seafood, insert a food thermometer into the thickest part. Safe temperatures are:

170˚ F for poultry (breasts)

180˚ F for whole birds

160˚ F for ground meat

160˚ F for pork

145˚ F for fish

Cheese

If you see mold on cheese and still want to salvage it, experts recommend cutting a full one-inch area around the mold. I recommend throwing it out; why take a chance?

Eggs

Raw eggs are a potential source for salmonella; when cooking eggs, cook them until the yolk is soft firm, not runny; always wash your hands after handling eggs. When making cookies, don't eat the cookie dough. Never let a child lick the bowl or beater when you're making a dessert with raw eggs in it.

The Bathroom

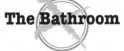

FACT! In a humid bathroom, a single bacterium can multiply to 1 billion overnight.

Soap

DANGER ZONE Use dispenser soaps because bar soaps can be laden with germs passed from person to person, not to mention they are slippery when wet. If you use bar soap, store it in a holder that allows it to air-dry.

Sponges and Scrub Brushes

That expensive loofah sponge you just bought is a nest for *Staphylococcus aureus*. Always dry it thoroughly after use. Disinfect it weekly with bleach and water.

STAPH AUREUS *can cause toxic shock syndrome, food poisoning, skin infections and wound infections.*

The Shower

My husband's grandmother was right: She used to insist that all grandchildren wipe her shower dry when they finished using it (a habit he's long since ditched). Wipe your shower dry after each use and spray it every few days with a mildew-busting product. Disinfect the shower once a week and always when someone is ill.

HOT TIP

OVER the Top?

"I wash my toothbrush with antibacterial soap before I brush my teeth." *Blatant with a capital B. Why not save yourself some time and invest in a toothbrush sanitizer instead?*

Toothbrush

Rinse your toothbrush under hot water for about twenty seconds after you use it and let it air-dry completely between uses. While most germs will be gone in twenty-four hours if the toothbrush dries completely, to be extra careful, dip it in Listerine (use a cup, don't just dip it in the bottle) or hydrogen peroxide and then dry. Communal toothbrush holders are a great place to share germs; if you use them, wash them in the dishwasher frequently. If someone in your house is sick, replace all toothbrushes just to be safe, because germs can survive in the warmth and moisture of the bristles. Store toothbrushes away from the toilet, preferably in a cabinet. Replace them every three months . . . long before they start to get grody.

The Sink

Disinfect it weekly; daily if someone is sick (especially the faucet handle).

A Germ Freak's ✓ GOTTA HAVE IT?

Violight Toothbrush Sanitizer. Voted one of the Coolest Inventions of 2004 by *Time* magazine, this high-tech toothbrush holder bathes your toothbrush with ultraviolet light, killing 99.9% of the germs and bacteria in ten minutes (it even turns itself off). It can hold up to four brushes, even electric ones. *www.violight.com*.

Towels

Have a separate towel and hand towel for each member of the house. If someone in the house is sick, use disposable paper towels made from recycled materials for the duration of the illness, unless you like doing laundry and want to wash cloth towels after every use.

Mouthwash

Drinking directly from that bottle is a definite no-no. To keep people from doing this, have paper cup dispensers, or individual cups or individual mouthwash for each person.

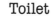

Toilet

"When we studied the aerosol effect of toilets, droplets were going all over the place—it looked like the Fourth of July."

Dr. Gerba

Always close the toilet lid before you flush. Disinfect the toilet bowl and lid weekly; more if you have children (or adults) who have accidents or if someone is sick.

A Germ Freak's ✓GOTTA HAVE IT?

The Magic John is a foot-activated toilet seat lifter that can be retrofitted for any toilet and installed in five minutes (or five hours if you're like me). Able to fit on round or elongated seats, it helps prevent germ transmission and makes it difficult for guys to find an excuse *not* to put the toilet seat down. *www.magicjohn.com.*

Bedding

Change your sheets once a week; daily if someone has a cold or flu. If you have young children who congregate in a family bed, fit your mattress with a waterproof pee-guard. Believe me, it's worth it.

Laundry

Because some germs can survive a laundry cycle, wash your underwear separately from other clothes. Use the hottest setting and use bleach or a detergent with bleach.

 Single men have lower bacterial counts in their living spaces than single women.

Dust

"There are lots of molds, bacteria and a wild assortment of tiny insect and animal parts that can be found within dust. Both **STAPHYLOCOCCUS** *and* **STREPTOCOCCUS** *bacteria can survive in dust for months at a time. Viruses that do not have a membrane may also survive in dust for long periods so it can easily be a source of potential infections."*

Jack Brown, Ph.D., *Don't Touch That Doorknob*

To reduce the dust in your home Paula Jhung, author of *Cleaning and the Meaning of Life*, offers these tips:

• Use the stove fan to suck up grease while cooking.
• Clean your air ducts. The first indication of dirty ducts is a fried dust odor when you turn on the heat or the air conditioner.
• If you live in a cold climate, reduce airborne soot in the winter

by burning well-seasoned hardwoods like oak and hickory instead of evergreens and packaged logs.

A smoker's home has twice the amount of dust as a nonsmoker's home.

- Houseplants, especially English ivy, Boston ferns and palms, can clean the air of some dust and bacteria. Don't overwater plants because wet soil can contribute to household mold. Don't buy fake plants, which only add dust. Who do you think you're fooling, anyway?
- Hardwood floor and areas without carpeting are less likely to spread dust and germs. Area rugs are better than wall-to-wall carpet because they can be washed. Since foot traffic brings in dirt, dust and grime, take off your shoes before you enter your house—it's much more comfortable anyway.
- Purchase a high-efficiency particulate-arresting (HEPA) filter that can remove pollen, dust, pet dander and bacteria.
- Cover air-conditioning vents with cheesecloth to filter pollen; use a HEPA filter if you have a forced-air furnace.
- If you have pets, bathe and brush them regularly to reduce dander.
- Purchase a good vacuum with an air filter that prevents the machine from recirculating germs. Think it can't happen? It can. According to Philip Tierno, Ph.D., in *The Secret Life of Germs,* one family kept suffering from stomach problems. After

some fact-finding they discovered that their vacuum cleaner kept recirculating salmonella into the air.

The Self-Cleaning Steel Home

Simi Valley, California, is home to the Landrys—and the nation's first antimicrobial home. After suffering damage to their previous homes from termites and earthquakes, the Landrys wanted a home that would be structurally sound and healthy for Mrs. Landry's asthma.

Built by AK Steel, the 11,000 square-foot home sits on 130 acres. It was built using about 200,000 pounds of steel, 35,000 pounds of which are coated with the antimicrobial compound AgION, which reduces fungus, bacteria and mold growth.

The coated steel is used in high-traffic areas as well as in the heating, ventilation and air conditioning systems. And if that doesn't make you want to go out and get a home like this, the kitchen features eight sinks, two cooking ranges and three dishwashers. Hmm, just like my kitchen . . .

At Work

"Because some cold and flu viruses
can survive on surfaces for up to 72 hours,
an office can become an incubator . . .
Even if someone goes home, the virus they
brought with them can linger. In fact, even after
72 hours, 700 viral particles of the cold virus
[can remain], enough to potentially
sicken seven people."

DR. GERBA

It's Monday morning and you're back in the office (at least physically). After putting your lunch away and getting coffee, you fire up your computer and officially start your day. The problem? You've already encountered 1,000 viral particles and you haven't done anything productive. What's the solution if you want to survive until quitting time?

Since HR rejected your memo to allow you to work in a hermetically sealed cube, this chapter reveals the germiest places in typical workplaces and outlines specific germ avoidance tactics for certain people.

Germ Hot Spots

You might think that your office desk is so clean you can practically eat off it—and some days you probably do. But truthfully, you'd be better off eating your turkey wrap from the toilet seat instead. According to a study conducted by Dr. Gerba, the average office desk harbors 400 times more bacteria than the average toilet seat.

"For BACTERIA, *a desk is really the laptop of luxury. They can feast all day from breakfast to lunch and even dinner. . . . A small area on your desk or phone can sustain millions of bacteria."*

Dr. Gerba

Surprisingly, bacteria levels on private surfaces, like phones and desktops, were higher than on photocopiers and toilet seats. Since you consider yourself to be fairly clean, how did your office get so germy? Usually it's from other people who directly contaminate your space or germs that hitch a ride back on your hands. The good news? Disinfecting these areas once a day can decrease bacterial levels by *99 percent or more*, even in the most contaminated spots.

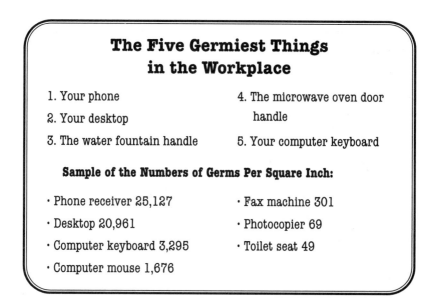

**The Five Germiest Things
in the Workplace**

1. Your phone
2. Your desktop
3. The water fountain handle
4. The microwave oven door handle
5. Your computer keyboard

Sample of the Numbers of Germs Per Square Inch:

- Phone receiver 25,127
- Desktop 20,961
- Computer keyboard 3,295
- Computer mouse 1,676
- Fax machine 301
- Photocopier 69
- Toilet seat 49

Try these tips:

- Disinfect your phone, including the mouthpiece and the number pad, and your computer keyboard and mouse.
- If you eat at your desk, disinfect the surface before. Don't take a working lunch because you'll be touching your food, your dirty pen, your food, your dirty Wite-Out, your food, etc.
- Bring your own bottled water, but make sure you're not toting around germs with it. Reporter Leslie Siegel collected bottles from five people and took them to Superior Laboratories in Reynoldsburg, Ohio, where they were tested for bacteria, mold and yeast. All five of them exceeded the EPA's limits for overall

bacteria in safe drinking water by *hundreds of thousands* of organisms.

 Get a new water bottle every time yours is empty or rinse it thoroughly under soap and water for at least thirty seconds.

• Oh yes, and . . . wash your hands!

Do You Recognize These Stealth Germ Spreaders?

The Martyr: She proudly professes that she's "never missed a day of work" despite coming in with pinkeye and infecting half of the office. Keep your distance from this Typhoid Mary.

The MIS Person. While he may delete viruses on your computer, he could be leaving one on your keyboard as he makes his after-hours' fixes. Yes, he can hack *into* any computer, but is he hacking *onto* yours? Make sure you disinfect your keyboard and phone after any upgrades.

The Wanderer. She loves to roam around, answering her pages from other people's phones. Don't let her use yours. Tell her you're sick or waiting for an important three-way conference call.

The Close-Quarters Cougher. You're stuck in a closed-door meeting and the person next to you is goose coughing . . . again. Quote some drivel from the *One Minute Manager* and wrap things up quickly. Ditch the coffee you brought with you, and oh, yes, wash your hands.

> **The "It's Just Allergies" Cougher.** A cough is a cough is a cough. A germ is a germ is a germ. Stay A-W-A-Y from this Phlegm Fatale.
>
> **The Hydrophobic.** Her fear of water manifests itself by her avoidance of the bathroom sink. Don't touch where she's touched.
>
> **The Spitter.** While the name speaks (or sputters) for itself, your best defense is to practice Strategic Seating at meetings and never sit within three feet of this person.

 The world record for sneezing is held by Donna Griffiths of Worstershire, England, who sneezed for 978 days in a row, stopping on September 16, 1983. Wouldn't you just love to share an office with her?

Hi Ho, Hi Ho, It's Off to Work I Go
... or Not

 33% of employees surveyed in 2003 said they worked while sick because of their workload; 26% said it was "too risky" to take time off; 18% saved their sick days for when their kids needed them.

Employees take note: If you come to work sick, you're no longer viewed as a vital cog in the machine, but a bacterial bottleneck who could render an entire department useless. According to the *Harvard Business Review,* presenteeism costs companies $150 billion each year and now the bloom is off the rose: The idea of the hero worker has lost its luster. For instance, one woman went to work with a bad cold and found her office mates trailing behind with disinfecting wipes. One man went to work, fully recovered from his cold, yet still noticed a coworker scurrying from his office with a can of Lysol when he returned from a meeting.

"**PRESENTEEISM** *isn't an ideology, a doctrine or any other 'ism.' It's the opposite of absenteeism. It's the practice of coming in to work when you should be in bed."*

Ellen Goodman, *The Boston Globe*

It's not that sick people want to take down the company. Most people would love to stay home huddled under the covers, admiring the Get Well bouquet their boss sent with the thoughtful note: "Come back when you feel up to it."

But really, is this going to happen? The average number of paid sick days for U.S. workers is about five per year—hardly enough to go around. Since you can spread a virus the day before symptoms hit and up to seven days after, this leaves many people having to go back to work while contagious.

If ego or economics deem you must go to work ill, there are ways to contain the contagion. Quarantine yourself to your office as much as possible. Tell your clients and coworkers *up front* that you're sick and let them decide if they want to come near you. There's nothing worse than being the recipient of an eyebrow waxing and finding out the hard way (or the wet way) that the beauty technician hovering over you has a runny nose. Strictly follow proper Respiratory Etiquette and hang the sign on the following page on your office door.

Talk with your boss or HR department about setting up a flu-season sick policy to benefit the company: Could employees with colds work at home with laptops? Make up work on a weekend? Could you set up a buddy system to finish work for others?

Rhinovirus
Present:
I AM A
HAZARD
TO YOUR
HEALTH.

Brainstorms,
Not Rainstorms:
Please Cover
Your Sneeze

Sick Leave Reform

The National Partnership for Women & Families introduced a bill to Congress in the summer of 2004 that requires companies with fifteen or more employees to offer six paid sick days that can be used for the employee or family members. So far California is the first state to mandate partially paid sick leave. For more information, go to *www.nationalpartnership.org*.

And you thought the office couldn't run without you. On February 21, 1990, NASA was preparing to launch the space shuttle *Atlantis*. Unfortunately, astronaut John Creighton had a cold and was man enough to admit it. His illness delayed the launch for a week, costing NASA $2.5 million.

In a survey conducted by Opinion Research Corporation, when asked what people would prefer sick coworkers do if they can't stay home from work, 42 percent chose having the sick person wash his hands as often as possible. Staying away from other people came in second. However, a few people—obviously not members of the HR department—suggested a harsher solution for infected colleagues: send them to a special "sick room" for the duration of their disease. Nice!

When to Stay Home

When you have a fever

When your nose won't stop running

When you have a persistent cough

If you're vomiting or having diarrhea (Duh.)

When you have aches or chills unrelated to a Pilates class or menopause

When you need a day to destress (or attend Opening Day)

When you have a leftover sick day

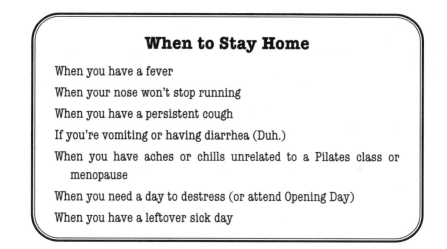

Waging Anti-Germ Warfare

In the winter of 2004, Massachusetts employers waged a war on germs. They installed antibacterial soap dispensers in company bathrooms (bad idea), hand sanitizers near community keyboards (good idea) and requested that sick employees stay home (best idea).

Miscellaneous Germ Avoidance Techniques at the Office

Don't Make Your Desk a Hangout for Germs

Do you keep a box of Kleenex on your desk? You're literally inviting a sick, germy person to blow her nose in your face. Keep your Kleenex out of sight. Also, if you're the go-to gal (yes, it's usually the females) for aspirin, Band-Aids and other necessities, you're inviting people with headaches and open wounds to use your workstation as triage central. Is this really a good idea?

OVER the Top?

"I always carry around a tissue in my blazer pocket so I can use it to open the bathroom door handles at work." *Good idea, as long as you lose the dirty tissue and get a new one each time you go.*

Don't Eat More Than You Planned On in the Cafeteria

The Coffeepot

The only thing worse than the person who takes the last bit of coffee and doesn't make more is the person who makes the coffee while contagious. Since most office coffee pots are rarely cleaned, bring your own coffee singles or buy coffee at Starbucks (think drive-through).

 60% of office coffee mugs have coliform bacteria on them; 10% of them have E. coli.

 E. COLI *can cause diarrhea, food poisoning and wound infections.*

The Refrigerator

Many Germ Freaks fear the fridge, but your food is safe if you bring it yourself. Make sure the fridge is in good working order so the food stays cold enough, and beware of sick poachers dipping into your stuff.

The Microwave Oven

The microwave door handle is one of the germiest items in the workplace, so wash your hands after you touch it and before you eat that pizza you just nuked. The microwave kills germs on the *inside*, but you're on the outside.

The Condiments

Steer clear of communal condiments. They could have been left out at room temperature for the entire week, and most have an illegible born-on date before *you* were born.

OVER the Top?

"I was on a special diet, so I bought several gluten-free and expensive salad dressings. Someone was dipping into them because each day more was gone. This person would leave the cover all crusty. One day I saw a black hair—not mine—stuck in the crust. Earlier that day I heard a woman hacking who had black hair. That was it; I poured the dressing in an opaque container and labeled it URINE SAMPLE. No one ever touched it again." *Most definitely blatant. Creative, too.*

The Doctor's Office

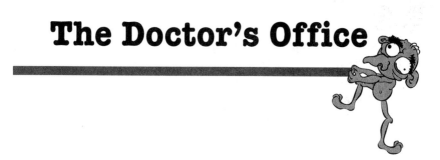

"Proper hand washing is an
enormously effective method of prevention.
I wash my hands before and after seeing
each patient in my office. I recently underwent
neck surgery. I'm more pleased that
my neurosurgeon scrubbed his hands
thoroughly than that he wore sterile gloves.
Hand washing is more important."

ALAN GREENE, M.D., FAAP

Doctor's offices are virtual petri dishes. Think about it: A group of sick people are forced to wait in a holding tank of contagion while their diseases commingle, mutate and reproduce. If you're just going for a "well visit," chances are you'll be sick by the time you leave unless you use these precautions:

- Schedule a first morning appointment. This way, the office has just been cleaned and not many people have been there to sneeze or slobber on the magazines, the door handles and the pen you sign in with. (Note to self: Bring my own pen.)
- If you have children, find a physician who has two entrances: a side for sickies and a side for well ones.
- Bring your own reading material and toys for your kids. While this will cut down on your germ load, it also saves you from reading last year's *People* and not noticing until page 93. In one very well-respected hospital, a plastic ball tossed back and forth among children spread Enterobacter, infecting all the kids who touched it. Remember to sanitize your kids' toys when you get home.

 ENTEROBACTER *can cause respiratory, urinary tract and other infections.*

- Never drink from any water fountains in doctors' offices!
- If you have kids, don't let them play on the floor (although this can be an impossible feat).
- If the physician leaves you waiting for a long time, don't try too hard to keep your kids quiet: if you let them emit a few ear-piercing screams you'll likely be taken to a more private room in the back sooner rather than later.
- Give your hands a very thorough decontamination when you get home.
- Change your clothes when you get home and put them in the wash.

Steer Clear of the Necktie

They've got you covered, how about them? A 2004 study by Dr. Steven Nurkin, a researcher at the New York Hospital Medical Center in Queens, showed that many doctors are sporting more than the latest neckwear. His team analyzed the neckties of forty-two doctors, physician's assistants and medical students as well as the ties of ten hospital security guards. The bad news: Doctors' ties were eight times more likely to contain germs than the guards'. The good news: None of the bacteria was resistant to antibiotics, and your doctor's just the one to write you a prescription.

A Germ Freak's ✓GOTTA HAVE IT?

Infectious Awareables, Inc., based in Encino, California, produces a unique line of disease-prevention products including ties, scarves and boxer shorts imprinted with colorful, magnified images of germs, from herpes virus (Oh, honey, you shouldn't have!) to anthrax bacteria (much more effective than a Dear John letter). In 2005, the company debuted Moi! The Humane Genome ("Wear yourself out!"). The company produced an award-winning video, *H.I.D.E. & S.E.E.K!*, that focuses on strategies for infection prevention. The company donates a portion of all sales to education and research of infectious disease. *www.iawareables.com.*

A Washed Pot Never Boils . . .

You're in the garishly decorated, depressingly outdated examining room, eavesdropping on the litany of complaints. "Yes, it's oozing more since yesterday." "What *color* is the phlegm?" "I'd say the stool is more runny than hard. . . ." As you wonder just how good the ventilation system is, the door flies open.

"Hello, I'm Dr. Nowashi, what brings you here today?" she asks, presenting her outstretched hand.

Did she or didn't she? If you find yourself in this situation, remember: It is your right to insist that all doctors wash their hands before examining you. It's not personal; it's your policy. While coming right out and asking a doctor if she washed her hands is a little uncomfortable, remember that more than 2 million Americans each year acquire infections in hospitals. According to the CDC, these infections cause 19,000 deaths directly, contribute to another 58,000 and are most frequently spread on the hands of health-care workers.

Real-World Maneuver:
Casually Asking the Doctor If He Washed

In order to avoid causing an awkward moment or diminishing the doctor-patient rapport, I interviewed some doctors who told me they have been asked on occasion by patients to wash their hands. They do not find it offensive, and it's not something they haven't heard before from administration. If you're still not sure, try these approaches:

Option 1: "I know this seems ridiculous but the last time I was in the [hospital], [my gynecologist's] or [the walk-in clinic]. . . . I got a bad infection. Can you please wash your hands before you start?"

Option 2: "I'm a great patient and I know we'll enjoy working together, but I really need you to wash your hands before you start your exam." (Say this in a happy tone and with a smile.)

More than twenty published studies have shown that alcohol-based hand rubs were much more effective than plain soap and water for reducing the number of live bacteria on the hands of health-care workers when used properly. It could be that your physician used one of those rubs before examining you. However, the evidence—and the fatalities—speak for themselves. Never assume. Always ask.

"There are some people, including physicians, who are quite antisocial in their behavior. During an eye examination I had an ophthalmologist who didn't wash his hands. I told him, 'You wash your hands before you touch my face.' As a patient you have that right."

Philip Tierno, Ph.D.

Researchers at the University of Washington conducted a study of how often medical personnel in intensive care units washed their hands. On average, only 38% did so as often as recommended. Many failed to wash their hands after changing dirty bandages or handling urine bags (yuck!). Respiratory therapists washed their hands about 70% as often as they should have; nurses and X-ray technicians about 40%. Physicians were the worst, washing less than 26% as often as recommended. Scary.

A Hand-Washing Hero

Ignaz Semmelweis, a medical student in Vienna in 1840, wondered why so many women who delivered babies in the hospital were dying while the richer women who had their babies at home with a private physician were not. Surmising that germs inside the hospitals were causing the disease, he discovered that medical students were passing the germs to the women because they went straight from the autopsy room after performing dissections to the maternity ward.

When Semmelweis rallied behind thorough hand washing, childbed fever became virtually nonexistent. So was Semmelweis given a Nobel Prize? A raise? Hardly. Semmelweis's physician-in-charge was either jealous or a jackass. He sabotaged Semmelweis's promotion and drove him out of Vienna, burying the hand-washing theory in the process. Childbed fever emerged again.

Sadly, Semmelweis died in an insane asylum at the age of forty-seven, distraught over the failure of the medical profession to accept his idea. Ironically, he died of an infection he got while performing an autopsy.

The Hospital

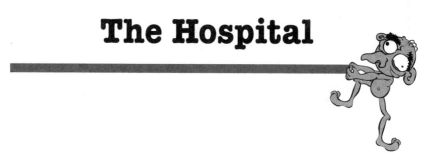

While the overwhelming majority of health-care workers should be commended for the work they do, when you enter the hospital you become susceptible to an onslaught of germs. While this book cannot cover all that you need to do to ensure a safe hospital stay, here are some basic tips. For a more thorough discussion, see some of the books in the Resources section.

- If you're having nonemergency surgery, ask that it be done on a Tuesday or Wednesday. In many hospitals the staff is sparse on the weekends, and Monday surgeries get moved due to spillover cases.
- Ask which pre-op tests you really need and why. Any time a needle has contact with your body, there's the risk of infection.

- Ask your doctor or surgical coordinator to compile a list of the drugs you'll receive in the hospital and why. When staff comes to your room to give you medicine, always ask that they check your chart and wristband.
- Ask if you can bank your own blood or have relatives and close friends donate blood for use.
- Ask your doctor if you'll need to take antibiotics and when. Surgical patients should receive antibiotics within sixty minutes of the procedure to reduce the chance of infection. A recent Medicare survey found that 44 percent of patients didn't receive the proper antibiotic treatment.
- Have someone you trust (preferably someone outspoken) be your advocate and watch over your care.
- Ask every staff member who touches you to wash his or her hands first. Artificial nails increase the chances that harmful bacteria will be transmitted to patients, so watch closely.

 Before hand washing, 73% of nurses with artificial nails had harmful bacteria present on their nails compared with only 32% of nurses without fake nails. These numbers dropped to 68% and 26%, respectively, after the nurses washed their hands.

Hand Sanitizers in Hospitals

In 2004, the CDC called on the nation's 5,700 hospitals to use alcohol-based waterless hand sanitizers. During an eight-hour shift in an intensive care unit, a nurse can save a full hour by using these instead of soap and water. Unfortunately, some hospitals are slow to install them, and in some areas, fire codes prevent their installation in hallways because they are alcohol-based and therefore flammable.

- If you have a catheter inserted, ask when it can be removed. The risk of getting a urinary tract infection increases when a catheter is left in for more than two days. If you feel any pain, request that the nurse check to see if it's clogged. Silver alloy catheters are a bit more costly to the hospital, but can prevent infections, so inquire if they use them.

- Tell your nurse if you have any pain or swelling in your arm or if your IV line gets clogged.

- If you're having major surgery, inquire about using a spirometer, a device that can help strengthen your lungs and reduce your risk of contracting pneumonia.

- If something doesn't feel right about your care, trust your instincts and speak up. This can be something minor or major. For instance, one woman who was never a Germ Freak was waiting for her daughter to wake up from invasive surgery. She watched as a janitor came into the sterilized room and tried to mop up the floor with a bucket of filthy, black water. She promptly told him to stop. She spoke to the nurse manager on duty and made sure the room was properly cleaned.

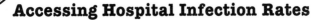

Accessing Hospital Infection Rates

Beginning in 2006, the public will be allowed to view hospital safety records for the state of Florida. Included in this information will be whether or not a hospital administered a required dose of antibiotics within sixty minutes of patients' operations. Later in 2006, the state will release how many people acquired infections at individual hospitals. Florida is one of the first states to release hospital infection rates, unfortunately not because of genuine concern, but because of a law passed in 2004.

The Supermarket

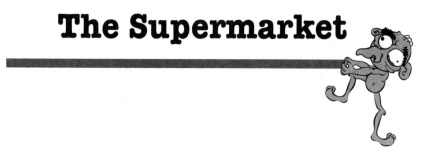

"Of all the consumer contact points in the
supermarket . . . shopping carts are the dirtiest.
Shoppers touch the carts as well as cough
and sneeze on them. Small children soil them.
As a result, E. coli and staph get transferred
from cart to customer or cart to groceries.
I cringe every time I notice a toddler
chewing on the cart's handlebar."

MARTIN SLOANE, "THE SUPER SHOPPER" SYNDICATED COLUMNIST

While there are very few of us who actually enjoy grocery
shopping, would knowing you could be picking up numerous
pathogens along with your staples make you dread it more? When
walking around those aisles, a Germ Freak's gotta be on high alert.

Attention Shoppers, There's a Special on E. Coli in Aisle 3 . . .

Shop at Off-Hours

Especially during cold and flu season. Don't shop on a Saturday or Sunday afternoon—it's double the people, double the germs (and triple the time). Plan ahead so you avoid shopping the day before a major holiday or before a big foodfest like the Super Bowl. And the biggest rule: Never, ever step foot in a supermarket the day they're giving flu shots—as soon as those automatic doors open, you can practically feel the cloud of contagion hitting you in the face.

DANGER ZONE

Clean That Nasty Cart

In America, shopping carts are not considered to be "food handling equipment" and therefore don't require strict levels of sanitation. A University of Arizona study revealed that shopping carts failed more hygiene tests than public restrooms: 54 percent of them contained bodily fluids and 21 percent of them tested positive for blood (!), mucus, urine (!) or saliva. Makes you think twice about sampling that deli turkey.

TIP Use a disinfecting wipe to clean the cart handle and wash your hands before eating anything in the store. If it's sunny, grab a cart from outside; the sun may have killed some of the germs.

✓GOTTA HAVE IT?

A Germ Freak's

The Clean Shopper. Invented by a mom, this award-winning shopping cart cover keeps babies and toddlers safe while shopping or out to eat. It has handy pockets to store toys and comes in a size for twins, too. And so Fluffy doesn't feel left out, they offer the Clean Pet Shopper, a shopping-cart cover for pets. *www.clean shopper.com.*

DANGER ZONE

Don't Graze

I cringe when I see people popping bulk produce or candy into their mouths while shopping. Not only are they stealing, they're potentially sampling the saliva of other people and then spreading their saliva onto everything they touch. Many kinds of produce and vegetables can carry diseases like salmonella unless they're thoroughly washed.

Choose the Ten Germs or Less Line

Always check out your checkout line before committing. Avoid cashiers who are sneezing, coughing or otherwise look sick. If someone directly behind you coughs, it's better to leave even the coveted number two spot in the express line than to stay and be hacked on while the woman in front of you struggles to find her coupons and then demands a price check on her 69-cent can of tuna.

Germ Freak Horror Story

"I went to the grand opening of an upscale health food store. As I walked through, I came to an olive bar where they had all of these gourmet olives. Just then I noticed this absolutely filthy man—he really looked like he was homeless—digging into a bowl up to his midarms, grabbing a handful of olives and then going back for more, without using a spoon. I went to the manager to tell him he had to do something to protect the health of the shoppers. If he wanted to do the charitable thing and feed this man that was great; but he couldn't have him double-dipping. He said he would take care of it. I went back to the store about a month later and who did I see? As I walked by the crock of soup available for sampling, the same man was scooping out a bowlful of soup with his cup—not the ladle. I will never go back to that store after the soup incident. I wrote the president of the company and never heard back."

Queasy Germ Freak

Watch the Meat Case

Most people touch several packages of meat or chicken before choosing the ones they want. If any blood leaked outside of the wrap and an employee wiped it without removing all of the germs, it can cross-contaminate your produce and fruit.

Shop for meats after you buy everything else, and keep them separate from the produce and fruit, even on the conveyer belt. Always put your produce in bags, and consider bagging your meat, too.

HOT TIP or OVER the Top?

"Keep your eye on the butcher. Is he putting on gloves and then running into the back room to get something with the same gloves on, then touching a few things before grabbing your turkey? When this happens, always ask him to put on a new pair of gloves." *Good tip if you like your deli meat sodium- and disease-free.*

"I went shopping one night, and the store was empty. While checking out, I noticed the cashier at the register next to mine had a raging cold: Her eyes were tearing, her nose was red and runny, and she kept wiping her nose with a tissue. She was bored, and instead of staying at her register and keeping her germs confined, she walked into my row, sneezed and then proceeded to 'help out' by straightening up the candy rack—which looked fine, by the way—and getting her germs all over the Tic Tacs. She came over to me and said, 'I'll help you bag.' I said, 'No, thank you. I like bagging.' She looked at me like I was a total control freak (Germ Freak maybe). But I don't want her sneezing on my blueberries that cost four dollars a pound."

Self-Bagging Germ Freak

The Public
Bathroom

"You know those little paper protective
bands that they put on toilet seats?
I don't trust those. I have a bit of a germ thing,
actually, but I don't let people see it."

TONY SHALHOUB, ACTOR, *MONK*

"Honestly, toilet seats get a pretty bad rap. . . .
People's hands—not backsides—transmit germs."

DR. RICHARD OLDS, INFECTIOUS DISEASE SPECIALIST,
MEDICAL COLLEGE OF WISCONSIN

The Port-a-Potty at a chili cook-off; asking for—and unfortunately getting—the key that opens the world's nastiest gas station
bathroom; the changing station at Chuck E. Cheese's after a few

explosive diapers—these bathroom atrocities are the stuff that can keep Germ Freaks up at night.

Germ Freaks aside, one thing most Americans have in common is an aversion to public restrooms and an arsenal of personal germ avoidance tactics we employ when we visit them. The good news: Some of our strategies actually work. The bad news? Some of the contact points we think are germy aren't that bad (the toilet) while others (the sink) are stealth germ-breeding grounds. Try these tactics so that you're not the one in five people who leave public bathrooms with fecal coliform—or worse—on their hands.

* 48% of women cover public toilet seats with paper guards
* 15% of Americans use tissue to turn faucet handles
* 14% of Americans avoid public restrooms altogether (these people are the anatomical minority, blessed with very large bladders)
* 8% flush public restroom toilets with their foot instead of their hand
* 2% use their elbows or wrist to dispense paper towels or soap

The Ten Commode-ments
of Surviving a Public Restroom

1. Choose Door #1

When choosing your stall, go for the first one. The middle stall in most public bathrooms is the germiest; the first stall is usually the cleanest. If you have the option, choose a bathroom with more than one stall, since more bacteria build up on a single stall.

HOT TIP *or* **OVER the Top?**

"I always use the handicap stall because it has less people, less germs." *Yes, they're cleaner, but are you ready to abandon your social etiquette for your hygiene? Better check page 44 to see if you are approaching the need for a Germ Freak Intervention.*

2. Check Your Seat

You shouldn't need too much help here: Don't sit on a toilet that's clogged or one that smells absolutely vile. Do a quick visual to make sure there's nothing crawling on the seat or any telltale urine drips.

3. Notice the Roll

Is there toilet paper? Is it dry or wet with who knows what? Never take a roll of toilet paper that's sitting on the floor (bathroom floors are loaded with germs). If you find an unopened roll of toilet paper in the stall, use it even if there's some left on the dispenser. Someone will finish the old roll; it doesn't have to be you.

4. Don't Squat

Remember: You are a human, not a hovercraft. The practice of "hovering" or squatting over toilet seats should be reserved only for those people who can guarantee perfect aim every time. There's nothing worse than plopping your butt down only to soak up someone else's urine. If this happens, don't freak out—you might fall off the seat, which is not only embarrassing, but a hygiene disaster. Sitting on someone else's urine will make you want to gag, but it shouldn't make you sick (urine is virtually sterile).

Germs of Endearment

Despite what your college boyfriend told you, you can't catch an STD from a toilet seat. "Generally toilet seats are not an issue when dealing with the microbes . . . of sexually transmitted diseases," said Charles Ebel, senior director of program development for the American Social Health Association. The association handles about 700,000 calls a year, many from gullible people who want to blame toilets instead of the real culprits.

5. Let Down Your Guard

What about our beloved paper germ guards? Do they work or are we just offending the person who left the stall immediately before us? Most experts say paper germ guards help your head more than your hiney. Many commercial paper guards are too thin, allowing liquid and germs to seep through. The guards can slip when you sit on them, and by putting one down—unless you drop it and let it flutter to the surface—you run the risk of touching the toilet with your bare hands. Better your fanny than your fingers. But no paper guard wastes more trees and clogs more toilets than the homemade wad-of-tissue variety. No MacGyver toilet covers, please! If you simply cannot give up using a toilet guard, make sure it's thick but still goes down the drain; it's bad etiquette to leave it on the seat.

 Toilets can send tiny drops of flying fecal matter 20 feet in the air when flushed.

6. Flush and Rush

"If you're using a public restroom where the toilet seats don't have lids, you should be prepared to exit the stall immediately after flushing," explains Philip Tierno, Ph.D. "The greatest aerosol dispersal occurs not during the initial moments of the flush, but rather once most of the water has already left the bowl." So, you have a good three seconds. Better to flush and rush than feel the gush.

7. Give the Foot Flush the Boot

The toilet handle is one of the germiest things in the public bathroom, so make sure you wash your hands thoroughly after touching it. While some coordinated Germ Freaks swear by the Foot Flush method, this isn't recommended. For one thing, you're putting your germy shoe on the handle. Secondly, accidents have been known to happen. Do you really feel like fishing your new flip-flop out of a public toilet?

 One-third of all Americans flush the toilet while they're still sitting on it—a nice way to get your butt wet and covered with E. coli!

8. Don't Dispense Germs

Go directly to the paper towel dispenser, but be careful. Don't use a wet section of paper towel because you can't be sure exactly what the liquid is. If a towel is wet, rip off the next one. Take the paper towel to move to step nine.

For Women Only

Sadly, ladies, we lose again. Not only do we have to wait twice as long to use the restroom as men, women's public restrooms have twice as much fecal bacteria as men's. Sanitary napkin holders are loaded with germs, so wash your hands well if you touch one. Never put your purse on the bathroom floor or the toilet tank: Use the hook or hold it.

9. Get Past the Sink

The hot water faucet is one of the most contaminated places in the restroom (the sink is the worst). People contaminate the faucet with dirty hands, and the water from the sink provides the perfect breeding ground for germs to grow.

Use a piece of paper towel to turn on the faucet; more importantly, when your hands are clean, turn off the faucet with the paper towel before drying your hands.

In a 2003 phone survey by Wirthlin Worldwide 95% of people said they wash their hands in public restrooms. Guess what? 55% of them were lying. Only 40% of people wash their hands after using the restroom.

Use Them or Lose Them: Hot Air Dryers

Lose them. Hot air dryers may be environmentally friendly, but not for your internal environment. These dryers pull air from the bathroom floor, not from the outside, so all they're doing is shooting a blast of hot bacteria full force onto your hands. One study showed that using electric dryers increased bacteria levels on hands by 162%! Better to drip-dry.

Germ Freak Horror Story

"I once saw someone put her toothbrush directly under the towel dispenser next to the sink. While she was in the bathroom, two people washed their hands right next to her toothbrush. Some of the water splashed on her toothbrush and then one of them pulled down the toweling right over her toothbrush. . . . I told her what happened and she looked at me like I was crazy. A few days later, she was sick."

10. Don't Touch That Knob

In a utopian Germ Freak society, everyone would practice good hygiene—at the bare minimum, they'd wash their hands correctly after relieving themselves. (See Hand Washing 101, page 21). But alas, we don't live in a perfect world. Testing done by John Pisani, Ph.D., a microbiologist at Micrim Labs, showed that bathroom door handles were loaded with *staph aureus* and other germs. Since the inside knob has *less* germs than the outside one, just imagine what is waiting out there. Use the Exit Strategies outlined on page 16.

A Germ Freak's
✓GOTTA HAVE IT?

Uri-Mate Protector. Individually wrapped urination funnel with a patented sloped design that gives women a clean and comfortable way to use public restrooms and unsanitary facilities. *www.urimate.us.*

CleanSleeve. The CleanSleeve was invented by a dad who was tired of holding his potty-training toddler above dirty public toilets. The plastic sleeve covers any U-shaped toilet seat. It's FDA approved, hypoallergenic to sensitive skin, and has been proven to stop not only wetness from passing through but has stopped radiation from being passed back to the seat from patients treated with radiation. *www.cleansleeve.com.*

Hygen-A-Seat. The Rolls-Royce of toilet protection, the Hygen-A-Seat is a portable, folding plastic toilet seat that zips up into its own germ-tight envelope. It comes in eight colors; a shoulder carrying case is also available. The Hygen-A-Seat motto: "If you don't touch it, you can't catch it." Amen! *www.hygen-a-seat.com.*

HoverSeat, aka The Stay-Dry Toilet Seat. Hopefully coming soon to a bathroom near you, this seat helps women (and men) "hover" (semi-stand/semi-squat) over the toilet in public restrooms. According to the patent application, it will prevent both "dribble-down" and "splash-back." Inventor Mindy Machanic explains: "The user stands by the toilet as usual, then starts to sit as usual, except that the seat helps the user stay hovering several inches above the bowl, with only two small squares on the back of the legs touching the supports. Add-ons and jazzy extras include special paper protectors for those who find even two small areas of seat to be unsanitary, and handle supports." For more information email: *hoverseat1@mindy-mac.com.*

There are the Oscars, the Emmys and the Addys. And, for the world of restroom sanitation, there's the Best Restroom Contest. Each year, with much fanfare (okay, so there's not much fanfare), Cintas Corporation honors companies "who go above and beyond the call of duty to present a pleasant, even memorable experience in a public restroom." The general public can vote online at *www.bestrestrooms.com*. Winners are awarded in April of every year. How tough is the competition? A prior runner-up, Wall's Automatic Pilot Toilet, in Boston, features self-cleaning toilet bowls and floors that are sanitized after every use.

The Final Word?

The World Toilet Expo is "the" show where key decision makers meet to improve sanitation worldwide and attendees can view the latest innovations and emerging trends in the international toilet industry. With forums including Toilet Culture and Nation Building; Cultural Distinction Between Reading and Creativity in Toilets; and Enhancing the City's Living Environment with Good Toilet Etiquette, it's no wonder the lines of attendees "back up." Hopefully most presenters don't get flushed before they speak. Who gets the dubious honor of being the number-two speaker?

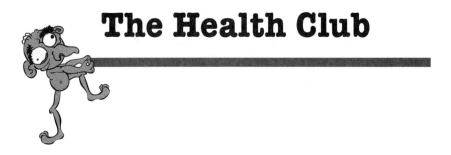

The Health Club

"The gym is an unusually effective place for the
transmission of germs. All those people, all that
exposed skin and all that sweat, can create a perfect
storm for spreading infections. . . . Spas, saunas
and showers in health clubs should all be posted:
'User beware; people deposit germs here daily.'"

PHILIP TIERNO, PH.D.

It's the ultimate irony: Some things you do to stay healthy
might just take you down. We all know those alfalfa sprouts you
struggled to stomach are a home to salmonella (hooray, you can go
back to that burger for lunch). Now we hear that when we go to the
gym to prolong our lives, we may be picking up germs that could do
us harm.

In January 2005, Philip Tierno tested several New York City health clubs for germs on *Primetime*. What he found wasn't pretty, and I'm not talking about the back-of-the-room view from a beginner's aerobics class. The investigation found nasty germs on the equipment and surfaces at several of the gyms.

The Equipment and Its "Health Benefits"

Dumbbells. Staphylococcus, Streptococcus viridans, diphtheroids and E. coli.

STREPTOCOCCUS VIRIDANS *has the potential to transmit SARS, influenza and colds.*

Exercise bike. Candida.

CANDIDA *can cause yeast infections and thrush.*

Shower floor. E. coli in unbelievable quantities.

E. COLI *can cause diarrhea, food poisoning and wound infections.*

Apparently, health departments go to gyms even less than the average American does—only once a year unless they receive a specific complaint. There are millions of germs on human skin. When someone sweats, those germs come pouring off. Germs like heat and humidity to grow, so a gym is a bacterial biosphere for the buff.

Many germs wouldn't necessarily make someone sick unless they were heavily exposed or immune compromised, so clearly the benefits to exercising outweigh not exercising, but the next time you go to the gym, try these tips:

1. Use a disinfecting or sanitizing wipe before you use a machine or piece of equipment. If your health club supplies the solution, make sure it's a disinfecting or sanitizing solution or it won't kill germs. Use a paper towel instead of the same rag that's been used by twenty other people.

2. Don't touch your eyes, ears, mouth or nose after touching the equipment.

3. Use a clean mat instead of lying on the carpeted floor.

4. Wear loose-fitting, breathable clothing (like cotton) instead of tight-fitting restrictive fabrics. Consider wearing long workout pants instead of shorts, especially if you have a cut.

5. Wear flip-flops in the shower.

6. Don't let anyone use your towel.

7. Bring your own soap for showering. Use pump dispensers instead of bars of soap for washing your hands. If you live very close to the gym, consider being stinky for a bit and use your shower at home.

8. Use an antifungal powder on your feet after you shower; air out your sneakers between workouts; get a new pair once your sneakers are smelly and worn.

9. If you wipe your face with a towel, don't use the same towel you used to wipe equipment down. Bring a backup towel for your face.

10. Never store damp or wet workout clothes in your locker or gym bag. If possible (it's usually not), rinse and hang your clothes up to dry before cramming them in your locker. Take them home every night and put them in a hamper to be washed.

11. If you like to take saunas, always sit on a clean towel. It's a fungal farm in there.

 You can catch crabs—otherwise known as pubic lice—from a sauna.

Stealth Germ Spreaders at the Gym:
Do You Recognize Any of These People?

Some of these familiar strangers you see most days may amuse
you, some may bug you and some may give you a bug when you
cross their paths. Can you separate the germ spreaders from
the non–germ spreaders?

Very Pepé Le Pew. He's raring to go and you can smell him five
feet away. Since it's obvious he doesn't own a stick of deodor-
ant, you question his other hygiene habits. You notice he sports
the same blue shorts every time you see him, so unless he has
five of the exact same pair with a matching grime stain on the
back, he doesn't believe in washing machines either.
Classification: Germ spreader. His shorts alone could be home to
millions of bacteria. Perhaps the gym members could pool their
money together and take up a New Pair of Shorts Fund?

The Spotter. You wonder if this guy actually ever works out
because he's always standing around asking everyone if they
need a spot. Before you take him up on his offer, make sure you
won't pick something up from him when he picks up your weight
from you. Classification: Not a germ spreader, unless he has a
cold or the flu.

The Sweater. This poor woman is sweating before she gets on a
machine. After her ten-minute bike session, water is spewing
from every crevice and the telltale puddle on the treadmill lets
you know her workout's finished. Classification: Germ
spreader. Germs love moisture. If she doesn't mop up, be sure
you do.

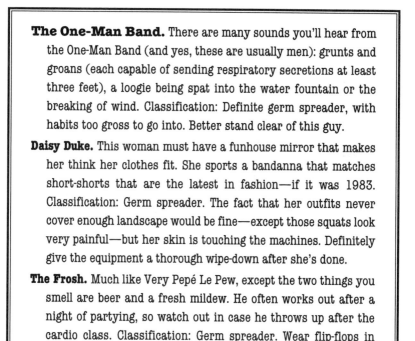

The One-Man Band. There are many sounds you'll hear from the One-Man Band (and yes, these are usually men): grunts and groans (each capable of sending respiratory secretions at least three feet), a loogie being spat into the water fountain or the breaking of wind. Classification: Definite germ spreader, with habits too gross to go into. Better stand clear of this guy.

Daisy Duke. This woman must have a funhouse mirror that makes her think her clothes fit. She sports a bandanna that matches short-shorts that are the latest in fashion—if it was 1983. Classification: Germ spreader. The fact that her outfits never cover enough landscape would be fine—except those squats look very painful—but her skin is touching the machines. Definitely give the equipment a thorough wipe-down after she's done.

The Frosh. Much like Very Pepé Le Pew, except the two things you smell are beer and a fresh mildew. He often works out after a night of partying, so watch out in case he throws up after the cardio class. Classification: Germ spreader. Wear flip-flops in the locker room.

Superbugs—Drug-Resistant Staph

The Centers for Disease Control and Prevention is increasingly concerned about a drug-resistant bacteria called *methicillin-resistant staphylococcus aureus* (MRSA) that's becoming more common, especially in athletic settings.

MRSA is the kind of germ scientists have theorized and worried about for years. Sixty-five percent of MRSA infections are drug resistant. Right now, MRSA is resistant to fifteen to twenty different antibiotics, so even if it's detected—which sometimes doesn't happen in time—doctors are left with limited treatment options. "Bacteria are unlike us humans. We have a generation time of about twenty-five years. They have a generation time of twenty minutes," explains Robert Daum of University of Chicago Hospitals. Within one day the superbug can mutate, becoming resistant to a different medicine.

Even more frightening, it can cause damage quickly. What begins as a minor cut, bruise or skin infection—things that many people might ignore or tough out—can become a deadly pneumonia or blood or bone infection in a matter of days. And in many cases, it's not being treated correctly. In fact, some patients with MRSA are worse off *after* seeing a doctor. The doctor gives the patient a weak antibiotic, which gives them a false sense of security and the germ more time to spread.

"In the scheme of public health threats, this has to rank close to the top," David Ropeik, director of risk communication at the Harvard Center for Risk Analysis, said of antibiotic resistance. "It's a serious threat now, and it's getting worse fast."

Even the NFL has been affected: Kenyatta Walker of the Tampa Bay Buccaneers and Junior Seau and Charles Rodgers of the Miami Dolphins reportedly were hospitalized with serious MRSA infections. Since 2000, there have been MRSA outbreaks at a fencing club in Colorado, among a college football team in Pennsylvania and high school wrestlers in Indiana.

Staying Safe from Staph

According to Dr. Luis Ostrosky-Zeichner, M.D., an infectious disease specialist at the University of Texas Medical School at Houston, you can take steps to help prevent staph infections. Any time you have a cut or skin breakdown, wash it with soap and water, keep it clean and dry, use antiseptic ointment, and keep it covered. The staph infection is contagious if the wound is weeping or draining, and if people share towels or other items that are contaminated. Wearing foot coverings in locker rooms and other commonly used areas can help prevent contamination. If the sore becomes unusually painful or red, get prompt medical attention. If red lines are present, get immediate attention because this is a likely sign that the infection is spreading.

And remember, it's always better to be safe than sorry.

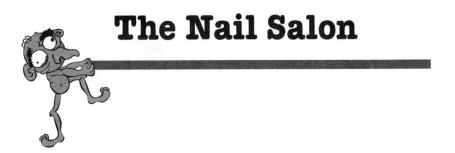

The Nail Salon

For many women—and growing numbers of enlightened men—a trip to have a pedicure is a relaxing experience. But disfiguring? Pedicure footbaths in nail salons have been found to have *Mycobacterium fortuitum,* a germ that can cause drug-resistant boils. In California, a nail salon infected more than one hundred customers, some so severely that they needed to be treated with skin grafts with medical bills topping ten thousand dollars. The culprit? A whirlpool footbath that became a bacterial soup when a dirty filter trapped hair, skin and organic matter. Yum.

Although nail salons are required by law to follow sanitary codes, many of them don't. A random investigation of nail salons throughout the country found that almost all of them tested positive for potentially harmful bacteria. But what can you do, short of not indulging? Since even Germ Freaks need their luxuries, follow these tips:

- The salon should look and smell clean; the staff should be neat and well-groomed.
- Tissues and cotton balls should be discarded after each client.
- As you're waiting for your session, observe your technician and see if she washes her hands and cleans the station between clients. She should place a clean towel over her table before each client.
- Your technician should wear surgical gloves.
- Pedicure baths should be disinfected after each client; your feet should rest on a clean towel.
- Your technician's license should be visible near her station; if not, ask to see it.
- Tools should be cleaned in a special sterilization product.
- The manicurist should apply a special disinfecting base coat to your nails.
- Ask whether your salon uses methyl methacrylate, MMA. It shouldn't. This is a cheap liquid adhesive that could lead to an allergic reaction, perhaps damaging kidneys and the liver. An indication that MMA is being used is an overwhelming smell that can make your eyes water when it's applied.
- Don't let manicurists cut your cuticles, because it's the cuticles that keep your nail beds safe from infections.

Nails longer than one inch are five times more likely than trimmed nails to carry pathogens that cause staph and yeast infections.

• Consider going au naturel, because acrylic nails increase the chance for a bacterial infection.

A Germ Freak's ✓GOTTA HAVE IT?

CutieKit. Several years ago, Valerie Moizel-Hatton contracted a small infection from unsanitary salon tools. Within one month, her nail fell off. Rather than swear off salons, she started bringing her own set of tools. Soon after, she met Laurie Shiers, a woman who had a similar nightmare experience. The two created a nail kit that people could take to the salons with them for some pathogen-free pampering. www.cutiekit.com.

Makeup Tips

5% of department store cosmetics are seriously contaminated with molds, fungi and other organisms.

• Never use the department store tester makeup. Always use a new disposable applicator when sampling products at a cosmetic counter. If that's impossible, request that the salesperson clean the item or the container opening with rubbing alcohol before applying it.

- Never share makeup.
- Throw away makeup if the color changes or an odor develops. Throw away eye makeup after three months.
- If you have an eye infection, throw away all eye makeup.
- Store makeup according to the packaging directions.
- If you have a cold or the flu and don't want to ditch your expensive lipstick, submerge it in rubbing alcohol for two minutes and scrape off the top layer. If you use Vaseline or cheap lip balm, throw them out after you've had a cold or flu and buy new ones.

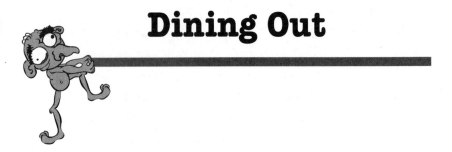

Dining Out

"The most shocking incidents are the
most blatant. Major infestations with insects
crawling on the walls during daylight hours. . . .
One local establishment—a big, well-respected
restaurant, doing thousands of dollars a day—
had no hot water for a week, until finally
a conscientious employee called us in."

ROBERT SOBSEY, WASHOE COUNTY PUBLIC HEALTH INSPECTOR

"What is the longest hair you've ever seen?" our
friend asked as we waited for our dinners to arrive.

"What do you mean? Like Cher or Lady Godiva?" I asked.

"I mean what's the longest free-floating hair that you've ever seen
off of someone's head?"

"What?!" I asked, waiting for the punch line.

"Look at your drink." There, wrapped around my glass was the longest, coarsest, blackest hair I'd ever seen. Forget the mystery of Sasquatch: he was behind the bar making piña coladas.

This story points to two facts: non–Germ Freaks love to make fun of us, and restaurants are not as pristine as you may think. As someone who spent many summers working in food prep and as a waitress, I know the restaurant reality. At times, kitchens are frenetic places where tempers—and hairs and sweat and Band-Aids—fly. If you eat out, you're probably taking in more hairs than you care to know about. The good news is, the hair itself won't make you sick. Unfortunately, it could be the canary in the coal mine that signals something rotten in Denmark—or in the walk-in fridge.

Whether it's a four-star restaurant or the burger joint down the street, there are four things to look for:

The Record. The local health department typically inspects restaurants once a year to make sure they maintain adequate kitchen facilities. The latest inspection score is posted in the restaurant or can be found online. Pay attention to word of mouth from friends, which is most reliable, and read reviews in newspapers. In general, established restaurants are usually in business because they haven't sickened their clientele.

DANGER ZONE **The Loo.** Before you sit down to eat, visit the bathroom: Is there hot water (any water)? Soap? Paper towels? If the answer is no, you should find another place to eat. No soap and water means the employees are not washing their hands before they make your food.

The Overall Appearance. Are the glasses dirty with lipstick stains or smudges? Are the utensils crusted with food debris? If so, the hot water may not be working or the staff is just plain sloppy. Get up and leave—or at least ask for a new glass.

The Table. The staff should clean your table with disinfecting spray and a disposable paper towel instead of a rag. If someone wiped your table with a dirty rag or sponge—which is the case at 90 percent of restaurants—clean the table yourself with a disinfecting wipe. Wiping your table is especially important if you have little kids who'll be eating half of their dropped dinner directly off of the surface.

 In 2003, 300 people got sick from salmonella, 150 of them seriously, when a Mexican restaurant in a Chicago suburb had no water to wash dishes or wipe tables due to a broken water heater.

OVER the Top?

"Whenever I order french fries, I eat down to the part my finger touches and then throw away the part my finger touched." *Over the top; have you considered using a fork?*

Finer Dining

In general, finer restaurants are apt to pay their employees more and train them more thoroughly in proper food handling and service. However, they're also apt to be handling your food more while preparing it. Here are three basic rules:

Keep It Simple, Stupid. In general, the simpler the preparation, the better. Several years ago I went to a very upscale restaurant that got rave reviews. Wanting something more elaborate than my usual grilled fish, I ordered a shrimp and scallop quesadilla with cheese, sour cream and spices. It was delicious. My mother-in-law also had a fish dish in a fancy cream sauce. We both got up at 2 A.M. She spent the next hour throwing up. I spent the night with severe stomach cramps. Obviously they didn't keep their fish at the proper temperature. If we had ordered our fish grilled, plain and simple, we probably (hopefully?!) would have been able to smell or taste that something was amiss. You can always order the sauce on the side.

Germ Freak Pet Peeve: Overhandled Food

"While most people oohh and ahh when their plate is drizzled with a raspberry coulis and their matchstick veggies are criss-crossed in a color-coordinated pattern, I'm just praying the person leaning over my dinner didn't have a runny nose."

A Meat-and-Potatoes Germ Freak

Go for Their Specialty. If you go to Jack's World Famous Crab House and order the chicken parmigiana, you can be sure that your entree isn't flying off the menu—or their delivery truck—as often as the signature crab legs. If you want authentic parmigiana, go to an Italian restaurant.

 Check Out Your Server. Wait staff have a tough job and don't get paid enough for what they endure. They also rarely get benefits or paid sick time, which means that server who has a bad cold probably can't afford to stay home. If your server looks sick or is sniffling, ask to sit in another station.

Ordering Tips from Anthony Bourdain

No restaurant-going Germ Freak should be without the book *Kitchen Confidential*, although you may want to wait to read it until after you've splurged at your favorite spot. Here are five tips from the book:

1. "I don't eat mussels in restaurants unless I know the chef personally. . . . More often than not, mussels are allowed to wallow in their own foul-smelling piss in the bottom of a reach-in."

2. "Bacteria love hollandaise. . . . Most likely, the stuff on your eggs was made hours ago and held on station. Equally as disturbing is the likelihood that the butter used in the hollandaise is melted table butter, heated, clarified and strained to get out all the bread crumbs and cigarette butts. . . . Hollandaise sauce is a veritable petri dish of biohazards."

3. "I never order fish on a Monday. . . . I know how old most seafood is on Monday—about four to five days old. . . ."

4. "Rested and relaxed after a day off, the chef is going to put his best foot forward on Tuesday; he's got his best-quality product coming in and he's had a day or two to think of creative things to do with it. He wants you to be happy on Tuesday night. Saturday, he's thinking more about turning over tables and getting through the rush."

5. "Brunch menus are an open invitation to the cost-conscious chef, a dumping ground for the odd bits leftover from Friday and Saturday nights or for the scraps generated in the normal course of business."

"If [a waiter] is sneezing and sniffling, not only would I change stations, I'd change restaurants because he's contaminated the whole place. If he's sneezing and dribbling, management should send him home."

Philip Tierno, Ph.D.

One Last Thing

Ditch the Doggie Bag. After your entrée was cooked, placed on a warmer, served, half eaten and left unrefrigerated while you made small talk and drove home, the bacterial count was climbing. In general, you have about ninety minutes from the time food is served to get it into your fridge. If you must, reheat leftovers to 160° F and eat them within twenty-four hours.

Fast Food: We'll Make You Sick in Less Than Five Minutes or Your Next Meal Is Free

"I have seen employees come right onto their shift and start making burgers without putting gloves on."

FAST-FOOD EMPLOYEE

If you watched the *Dateline* report "Dirty Dining," even the delectable scent of french fries probably couldn't get you back into a fast-food place—for a few months, anyway. *Dateline* investigators found, among other things: a dead rodent decomposing in a rat trap, a worm in a salad (no, worms don't count as protein on Atkins), a cockroach in a soda and gum in a taco. What's a Germ Freak to do? As with other types of dining, there are some things you can look at before you decide to place your order:

- Is there soap and water in the bathroom?
- Is the staff wearing gloves to prepare the food?
- Are they using tongs to get ice?
- Is anyone eating while preparing food (they shouldn't be)?
- Are the plates at the salad bar chilled? Is ice surrounding the items?
- Is the staff wiping surfaces with dirty rags instead of paper towels?

If you see one of the above behaviors, eat with caution. If you see two or more, turn around and leave.

Germ Freak Pet Peeve:
Nasty Play Areas

I took my kids to the play area at a fast-food place. As soon as I walked in I could tell it reeked of urine. I gave them the benefit of the doubt thinking maybe a kid just had an accident. The next week we went back and it smelled even worse. I will never go to that restaurant again.

Buffets:
All-You-Can-Eat Germs for $6.99

I only eat at buffets if I have to. There are too many people who double-dip, stand and graze or fog up the germ guard barrier trying to get a better look. I also know that buffets are a low-cost way to cleverly disguise food that didn't sell as its original incarnation. That quiche you're eating has had more lives than Shirley MacLaine. If you just can't pass up a good deal, at the very least pass on these buffet monstrosities:

1. **Chicken, Shrimp or Tuna Salads.** These salads are almost always made from old chicken or fish, which significantly increases the chance of foodborne illness. Mayonnaise kept out too long is never a good thing.

2. **Bacon or Sausage.** It's too risky to eat these foods if they're not kept hot enough or the buffet does not have a high turnover. Due

to the massive amounts of salt and additives, it's hard to know if you're eating a spoiled sausage because they all taste the same.

3. **Jell-O Salads.** At least fifty germy kids took them up on their offer to "Watch it wiggle, see it jiggle."

4. **Oatmeal.** While the cheap made-from-water kind you're getting at a buffet doesn't spoil, it's too easy for an employee to see a wad of something in the middle and mix it in, with no one the wiser.

5. **Soups or Chili.** Are you sure these are piping hot? Even so, some employees don't clean out the crocks between uses but simply add more to the top and mix. Let's just say there's probably more of a cheese layer on the *bottom* of your French onion soup than the top.

6. **The Bread.** Seems safe, right? Well, just watch—no one ever uses the tongs.

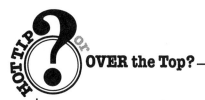

OVER the Top?

"I always wash my hands before and *after* I serve myself at a buffet. Many people don't wash their hands and then they touch the tongs. Or even worse, the dirty tongs that ten people touched are laying on the food." *Good tip, although if you keep going back for more, it could take you awhile to get out of there.*

Five Defensive Buffet-Line(Man) Moves

1. **Go early.** Don't go to the early bird buffet at 8 P.M. and expect to get food that hasn't been coughed on at least a few dozen times.

2. **Go deep.** Take your food from the back of the bin or way in the bottom. Likewise for your serving plate.

3. **Go fresh.** Avoid communal condiments kept uncovered on tabletops like cream, syrup, ketchup, pickles and mayonnaise. Made-to-order omelettes or stir-fries are safer; if you have the option, they're worth the extra wait.

4. **Go wide** around the grazers, gropers and double-dippers. Don't feel rude: They're rude to use the buffet as a trough.

5. **Go "cold turkey."** By law, buffets and salad bars must be kept at certain temperatures to keep food safe. Temperatures between 90 and 110° F breed bacteria that can cause food poisoning. Unless you have a thermometer in your pocket (kudos if you do!), look for chilled plates, ice around the items and a cold glass display panel.

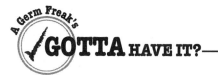

GOTTA HAVE IT?

Table Topper Stay-in-Place Mats are disposable adhesive place mats that stick to table surfaces, keeping infants and toddlers from eating their food directly off of dirty tables. With designs like ABC, Sesame Street, SpongeBob Square Pants and Dora the Explorer, they even keep your kids entertained, so you just may get to finish your meal while it's hot. *www.tabletopper.com.*

What most people call "stomach flu" or a "24-hour virus" is likely to be a mild food poisoning, usually from a common bacterium like salmonella or staphylococcus.

If you think you contracted a foodborne illness at a restaurant, contact your local health department. Many times, people will suspect the last meal they ate as the one that made them ill. This may not be the case. Most bacterial and many viral agents of foodborne illness can take between one and three days to develop or "incubate." By contacting your local health department, you could help stop an outbreak—and at least you get to vent.

Airports and Airplanes

"Have you ever wondered why the pages
of your in-flight magazine are sometimes stuck
together? On my last flight I saw a man in the
next row with a stream of snot coming out of his
nose. He couldn't find a tissue, so he reached into
the holder and got a magazine. He wiped his
nose and whipped the boogers onto the pages.
Then he closed it and put it back. Now I bring
my own magazines every time I fly."

A FREQUENT-FLYING GERM FREAK

Our trip from hell—fondly named this by me, my husband
and everyone within earshot of our 22-month-old-twins—began
like most flights do, at the airport with a three-hour mechanical

delay (the crew didn't show up). Not to fear. I had enough toys, snacks and sanitizing products to last a week.

Hour one: Quiet twins eating raisins, Mom Purelling their hands after they pulled trash out of the wastebasket, Dad commenting how great the kids are behaving (mistake).

Hour two: Well-behaved kids begin to whine; rolling on the floor officially commences; Purell, wipe, Purell.

Hour two and a quarter: Whining is now wailing; passersby shooting us The Look and hoping we're not on their flight; Purell bottle is empty.

Hour two and a half: Son licking the public pay phone; daughter lying headfirst on airport linoleum; Dad pretending he belongs to another family.

Hour three: The plane is fixed (the crew arrives). With three hours of travel time left, Mom is tempted to forgo hand washing before the kids eat their lunch . . . but I didn't do it. You must remain vigilant no matter how drained you are.

When traveling, it's easy to fall into complacency—just eat that hot dog on your layover or drink that airplane coffee that tastes like rocket fuel. Don't let a change in your routine lead to complacency, because airports and airplanes not only carry millions of people, they carry billions of germs.

A study by professor John Balmes and colleagues at the University of California at San Francisco, found that one in five people will get a cold one week after their flight—approximately four times the risk than if they had stayed at home.

Germ Hot Spots in Airports

• Always follow the Germ Freak guidelines for using public restrooms.
• Pack *lots* of instant hand sanitizer or disinfecting wipes. Clean your hands whenever you contact these germ hot spots: ATM machine, ticket counter, ticket counter pen, escalator handrails and public pay phone.
• Wear socks so you're not barefoot for the security check-in.

Airplanes: Germ Freaks at 30,000 Feet

Once you board the aircraft, staying safe gets simpler because there are only two rules to remember: Don't touch anything and don't breathe. There's a reason that a Germ Freak in row 5B cringes when someone coughs in row 7D. . . . It's only a matter of seconds until he or she is enveloped in a Chernobyl of contagion. Check out these facts:

• In 2003, twenty-two people contracted SARS on an Air China flight from Hong Kong to Beijing, a phenomenon researchers call "superspreading." The flight was three hours long, and individuals sitting seven rows away from the infected person were infected.

- In 1979, the CDC found that more than 70 percent of passengers on a jet delayed for three hours on the ground caught the flu from a fellow passenger. (Since 1995, ground delays have jumped 130 percent.)
- In 1996, a woman with drug-resistant tuberculosis took an eight-hour trip from Chicago to Hawaii. Afterward, nearly one-third of the people sitting within two rows of her tested positive for the disease.
- The CDC receives about a dozen reports a year of people who catch meningitis from sitting near infected people on airplanes.

The Dirtiest Travelers Exposed

An August 2003 study by Wirthlin Worldwide found that as many as 30% of travelers don't wash their hands after using public restrooms at airports. The study observed over 7,000 people at different airports. The results:

The Dirtiest

Chicago Men's Room: 38% did not wash

San Francisco Women's Room: 41% did not wash

The Cleanest

Toronto Men's and Women's Room: 95% and 97% respectively. (The Toronto stats may be attributed to the fact that people were more diligent since Toronto had just experienced a major SARS outbreak.)

Germs Don't Need Much Leg Room

A typical plane has only 1.5 cubic yards of space per person and recycled air; an outdoor stadium, by comparison, has 5 cubic yards of space per person and fresh air. On a typical narrow plane with 100 passengers, about five of the passengers will have a cold or flu. If the plane is arranged with seats of five rows across, the chances of you sitting close to the sick person are:

A. Very likely
B. Very likely
C. All of the above

Germ Freak Horror Story

"My family and I flew across the country on the day before Thanksgiving. Not long after we landed, my son started getting a runny nose and had a low-grade fever. *Not another cold!* I thought. He had been in day care and was constantly sick. Thanksgiving Day, he was very irritable and tugging on his ear. I called my cousin, an ear, nose and throat doctor, and asked him to prescribe some amoxicillin since I was sure this was an ear infection. My cousin didn't want to prescribe an antibiotic without seeing my son, but he did it and told me to keep a watchful eye on my baby.

"The next day, my son looked yellow and he was lethargic. Then he vomited. I knew something was terribly wrong. We rushed him to a local physician who could tell right away that something was wrong and sent us for blood work. They found that my son had pneumococcal meningitis—a bacterial infection that, if left untreated, is fatal.

"The doctors put my son on the strongest IV antibiotic they had. He was in intensive care for three days and then released for two weeks of home IV antibiotic treatment. Today, he is a happy, healthy six-year-old.

"The doctors said they don't really know how he picked up this infection (for which there is now a vaccination). I think flying on the busiest day of the year could have had something to do with it. Now I avoid flying during the really busy holiday times."

A Germ Freak Home for the Holidays

In addition to the flu, cold, TB and meningitis, other diseases that can be spread by high air recirculation or low ventilation include whooping cough, measles, mumps, chicken pox, shingles and infectious mononucleosis.

Tips from Frequent-Flying
Germ Freaks

Pick your flight. Choose flights that are less crowded or morning flights that have a lesser chance of being delayed or grounded. Avoid Boeing 757s because they don't have as much ventilation as Boeing 747s or 727s.

Pick your seat. Book a seat as far forward as possible. Studies show there's up to ten times more fresh air in the front of the plane so pilots stay awake. Air quality aside, the farther you are up front, the less people will be bumping into you and using your arm as leverage as they make their way to the bathroom (see page 137 for the gruesome details).

Pack your Purell. Chances are high that the traveler before you didn't wash his hands, so you need to wash yours. Use a hand sanitizer after touching these germ spots: the touch-screen TV, the call button, the air vent button, the instructions for exiting the plane (I know, no one reads these!), tray tables, magazines, windows, overhead bins, headphones, and, of course, the nasty bathroom.

"Airplane bathrooms are a disaster. Think about it: You've got two bathrooms for 100 people. The water almost never comes out more than a drip and you tend to touch many surfaces. In all of our studies we've found E. coli in every airplane bathroom on everything, including the faucets, the door and the sink."

Dr. Gerba

Avoid airplane pillows and blankets by bringing your own pillow or doing without. Due to rapid "cleanings" between flights, you could very likely use someone else's contaminated pillow that's been sneezed or drooled on within the past hour.

Would You Like Me to Fluff Your Blanket?

In November 2000, an airline service union accused the top airline laundry provider of not washing blankets or sanitizing headsets before sending them back to the plane. The laundry service employees claimed they were told that if blankets didn't "look dirty" to throw them in the dryer and "fluff" them up; they also said they were told to separate tangled headsets and repackage them without cleaning them. Samples from the headsets and blankets found traces of *Pseudomonas paucimobillis*, a bacterium that can cause eye and lung infections, and E. coli bacteria.

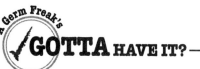

GOTTA HAVE IT?

The **Pocket Pillow,** a flannel case that can be stuffed with extra clothes and used as a pillow, or folded up to pocket size when not in use. *www.distantlands.com.*

Add a mask to your in-flight ensemble. If you're immune compromised, consider wearing a mask. In order to pull off wearing a mask, think "style," not "sanitation." Pretend you're Omar Sharif, or Barbara Eden in *I Dream of Jeannie.* When you are wearing your mask, some people will look at you like you're a freak. But trust me, they'll look even freakier next week when they've broken out in shingles. If you're feeling weird about the mask, try a portable air purifier.

Use a nasal spray before boarding (with your physician's consent) so your nasal passages aren't dry and susceptible to invaders. You can also coat your nostrils with vitamin E, food-grade olive oil or some Vaseline.

Single Germ Freaks: Forgo the last tip if you think your soul mate could be on the plane. There's no way in this lifetime that another Germ Freak will go near you with a shiny, goopy nose that from a distance looks like the beginnings of a rhinovirus. On the other hand, if he is a very serious Germ Freak, he will immediately "get you," and you two could spend hours—or a lifetime—sharing germ tips.

A Germ Freak's
✓GOTTA HAVE IT?

The **Air Supply Mini-Mate** Purifier is a small, portable device you can hang around your neck that kills chemicals, airborne germs and odors (great for when you get stuck near the bathroom). *www.pentex.com.*

The Air Right filter is a portable filter that you attach to the air vent over your seat, removing 99.5% of bacteria and viruses from your air space. Find it at airport stores or *www.airright.net.*

Don't fly when sick with the flu, a sinus or ear infection, a fever or even a bad cold. Not only will you get others sick, you can damage your health. If you're immune compromised, consider avoiding flying during flu season or peak travel times.

Don't complain about the pretzels. While many people lament that they used to get "a meal" with their flight, be happy with your three pretzels. Diana Fairechild, former flight attendant and author of *Jet Smarter*, explains: "Working over 10 million miles as a flight attendant, I have prepared and served countless airline meals. . . . I have been there when spoiled food was provisioned, food that had been dropped on the floor was served to passengers, ovens were inoperative so that the food served to passengers was not cooked properly, passengers and crew members have gotten sick from food poisoning. For these and other reasons, I recommend that passengers abstain from eating on board."

Don't drink the water. In January 2005, the EPA issued a statement that drinking water on planes may not be safe. After testing 169 planes at random, twenty-nine of them tested positive for E. coli bacteria. Don't request a cup of coffee or tea, which is made from the same water. Instead, keep yourself well hydrated with bottled water. Tim McCall, M.D., a specialist in internal medicine, recommends drinking eight to sixteen ounces of water or another noncaffeinated beverage the hour before you fly, plus a similar amount every few hours after lifting off. Of course, depending on the size of your bladder, this means you'll be visiting the nasty bathroom quite a bit.

"I stopped drinking airplane water my first year of flying after I saw floating particles in the water, and also after I saw mechanics filling the airplane water tanks from hoses on the runways wherever we landed—even Bombay."

Diana Fairechild, Former Flight Attendant, Author, *Jet Smarter*

According to an MSNBC poll:

77% of people wouldn't go near airplane water

15% of people would drink it but be concerned about its quality

8% think it's just fine

A fellow Germ Freak passed along this letter, which has been making the rounds of the Internet. We thought it was too funny (and true) not to share it. As far as we can verify, it is authentic.

Dear Continental Airlines,

I am disgusted as I write this note to you about the miserable experience I am having sitting in seat 29E on one of your aircrafts. As you may know, this seat is situated directly across from the lavatory, so close that I can reach out my left arm and touch the door.

All my senses are being tortured simultaneously. Its difficult to say what the worst part about sitting in 24E really is? Is it the stentoh of the sanitation fluid that is blown all over my body every 60 seconds when the door opens? Is it the wooosh ouf the constant flushing? OR is it the passengers a**es that seem to fit into my personal space like a pornographic jig-gaw puzzel?

I constucted a stink-
shield by shoving one end
of a blanket into the
overhead compartment -
while effective in blocking
at least some of the
smell, and offering a small
bit of privacy, the a** -on
-my-body factor has increased,
as without my evil glare,
passengers feel free to
lean up against what they
think is some kind of
blanketed wall. The next
a** that touches my shoulder
will be the last!

I am picturing a board
room full of executives
giving props to the young
promising engineer that
figured out how to squeeze
an additional row of seats
onto this plane by putting
them next to the LAV.

I would like to flush his head
in the toilet that I am
close enough to touch from
my seat.   , and taste,

Putting a seat here was a very bad idea. I just heard a MAN GROAN in there! THIS SUCKS!

29E

DEPICTION OF MANS BUTT IN MY FACE.

Worse yet, is I've paid over $400.⁰⁰ for the honor of sitting in this seat!

Does your company give
refunds? I'd like to go
back where I came from
and start over. Seat 29E
could only be worse if it
~~were~~ inside the bathroom.
was ~~located~~

I wonder if my clothing
will retain the sanitizing
odor.... what about my hair!
I feel like I'm bathing in
a toilet bowl of blue liquid,
and there is no MAN in a
little boat to save me.
I am filled with a deep
hatred for your plane designer
and a general dis-ease that

May last for hours.

We are finally decending, and soon I will be able to tear down the stink- shield, but the scars will remain.

I suggest that you initiate immediate removal of this seat from all of your crafts. Just remove it, and leave the smouldering brown hole empty, ~~for~~ a good place for sturdy / non- absorbing luggage maybe, but not human cargo.

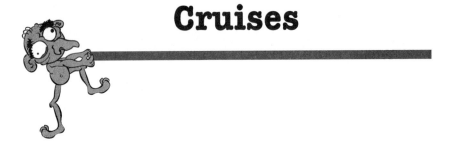

Cruises

"My boyfriend and I went on a seven-day cruise.
One little boy peed on the pool deck, and a little
girl threw up in the pool. Next time I would
get a boat with less kids and less germs."

CRUISING GERM FREAK

Getting sick on vacation is a real drag, especially when you won't get any more time off for 346 days and you spent so much money and excitement to get there. Being sick on a cruise is particularly unpleasant; it's no fun trying to hurl into a toilet when the boat is rolling and the small quarters are closing in on you. As a cruise passenger, the sheer fact that you're in an enclosed (albeit large) space with thousands of other people puts you at risk.

The good news: After the Norwalk virus gained media attention, it also got the cruise lines' attention. Across the board, cruise lines are taking extra precautions. Some cruises require passengers to pass through disinfecting stations when they reboard the ship, signs recommend that passengers wash their hands, stewards pass out disinfecting wipes to passengers when they grab their trays at the buffet, and on the high seas, the "forearm tap" has become a popular greeting instead of shaking hands. Hmm, makes a Germ Freak feel right at home. Here are some things you can do to stay safe on the high seas.

Check Out Your Ship

The formal way: To find out about a certain ship's sanitation record, go to the CDC's Web site (*www.cdc.gov*) to the Vessel Sanitation Inspection Report Green Sheet (*www.2a.cdc.gov/nceh/vsp/VSP_RptGreenSheet.asap*). A maximum score is 100 points, with 86 or higher judged as acceptable. The best way to get an accurate picture of a ship's sanitation record is to evaluate several of the ship's scores over a period of time.

Word-of-mouth: Log on to *www.cruiseopinions.org* to post questions and to read others' candid comments about particular cruise lines.

Check Out Your Destination

Research your cruising destination for any health concerns in that area. Seek medical advice six weeks before your cruise in case you require any medication or immunizations before you leave. Consider visiting a travel clinic near you through the International Society of Travel Medicine at *www.istm.org*. The CDC Web site also has a travelers section, which includes vaccination requirements: *www.cdc.gov/travel*.

Other Tips to Stay Healthy

- See the Restaurant chapter, since much of what you'll be doing on a cruise is eating.
- Many cruise lines offer extra-tariff restaurants with more intimate dining areas—more private dining typically means fewer germs.
- Dine al fresco when you can.
- If you don't have kids, avoid family-centered cruises. Try the more upmarket lines with smaller ships.
- When booking your cruise, avoid spring vacation weeks or the college spring break season.
- When eating away from the ship, choose foods and beverages carefully. Poor sanitation in some countries may lead to contaminated food and beverages. Be wary of undercooked or raw meat, raw or undercooked seafood, salads, ice and raw sprouts. Steer clear of street food vendors, especially if they serve fresh-cut fruits.

How Much of a Threat Is the Norwalk Virus?

The cruise industry has been hit hard—at least publicly—by the Norwalk virus, sometimes called norovirus. In January 2005 a Holland America ship had to end a cruise midcourse because more than 200 passengers were stricken with gastrointestinal illness. So should you avoid cruises?

Actually, you're less likely to get norovirus on a cruise than you would in your workplace, a school or another enclosed space. "The reason you hear about norovirus on cruise ships is because they are required to report every incidence of gastrointestinal illness. Nowhere else in the public health system of the United States is norovirus a reportable illness," explains David Forney, chief of the Vessel Sanitation Program.

23 million people—8% of the population in the United States—contract norovirus annually. Less than 1% of all cruise ship passengers are affected annually.

Cruise ships go through rigorous sanitation procedures that include disinfecting public surfaces—including door handles, elevator buttons and railings—and isolating anyone who is sick at the first signs of illness. Some cruises are offering incentives like discounted future fares to ensure sick people stay in their rooms.

"The most preventative measure people can take is washing their hands frequently," says Michael Crye, president, International Council of Cruise Lines. Crye said that after the last two years of outbreaks, he has a whole new appreciation for how easily germs spread. "Today I think twice about putting my hands on banisters in any public building. I think twice about pushing buttons on elevators. I think twice about doorknobs."

I hear ya.

Hotels and Motels

"The first thing you need to do is
remove that disgusting quilted comforter.
There's a reason they are so hideous looking:
it's to hide the dirt and stains! Just think of how
many naked people have sat on that comforter
and done who knows what on it. Remember Mike
Tyson's rape trial when they found body fluids
from prior guests on his hotel bedspread?"

TRAVELING GERM FREAK

The most important thing to remember when you travel is
that not everyone is as clean as you. Let's face it, some guests are pigs,
and the housekeeping staff is sometimes so busy that they can't clean
as thoroughly as they'd like (or you'd like). While the majority of

149

hotels do a good job with cleanliness, how can you be sure? For one, the price of the room is usually a good indicator. In one study, Dr. Gerba found a "statistically significant" relationship between a room's price and bacterial levels in a study of twelve Arizona hotels. The pricier the room, the fewer the bacteria. So live a little (literally!) and splurge on that fancy room. Then check the following areas, and you can sanitize the space in less time than it takes you to figure out how to work the TV (by the way, careful with that remote!).

- **The comforter/top blanket:** Take it off immediately when you get to your room and chuck it in the closet. Many hotel chains are replacing their dark-patterned comforters for light-colored duvets, knowing that most guests—not just Germ Freaks—don't trust the colored ones.

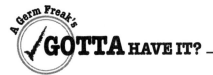

✓GOTTA HAVE IT?

Suspicious of hotel bedding? Pack a DreamSack, a sleeping bag-like sack that stuffs into its own 8"x4"x1" pouch. It keeps you cool and dry in the summer, and warm when it's cold. It's got a built-in pocket for a pillow and a side opening that closes with tab fasteners. Machine washable and quick drying. *www.magellans.com.*

OVER the Top?

"I always bring my own pillow, sheets and towels. The only thing I use the hotel towels for is to put on the floor so my feet don't have to touch the tile." *Middle of the road on number one; way over the top on number two.*

- **Three germ hot spots.** Disinfect the TV remote, the telephone and the refrigerator door handle. While these are frequently handled, they're rarely cleaned.
- **Pillows.** Do you really want to put your head on that pillowcase where someone else's drool has been? How much space or effort will it take you to pack your own pillowcase? If you don't want to do that, you can call housekeeping and ask them to deliver some additional pillows, taking the chance that these are clean.
- **Ice buckets.** There's a reason that these come with plastic liners. I have seen ice buckets being used for more than you wish to know. When a drunk fraternity brother feels the need to hurl, he's likely going to go for: 1) the toilet (if he can make it); 2) the wastebasket (if he can find it); or 3) the ice bucket. Even if someone hasn't done something nasty in it, housekeeping generally doesn't get around to cleaning these.

- **Coffeepots.** Most hotel staff don't wash the in-room coffeepots enough to stop germs from growing. Better to bring your own instant coffee, coffee single packets or go to a coffee shop. Really, has any hotel-room coffee *ever* satisfied your coffee fix?
- **Towels.** There's not much you can do about the towels except to pack your own. If you have a sunny patio or deck, hang them out in the ultraviolet light for an hour or so.

- **Tubs and showers.** While I personally don't wear flip-flops in the shower, I admire those who do. If you don't want to pack flip-flops, clean the tub with hot, soapy water or disinfectant spray. *Never* take baths in hotel tubs.
- **Cups and glasses.** Thoroughly clean the cups and glasses with hot water and soap.
- **Your toothbrush.** Be careful where you lay your toothbrush. Place it safely in your travel case after it's dry. The surrounding sink and countertop are not to be trusted.

48% of Americans check the cleanliness of their hotel before they unpack or turn on the TV.

Don't Let the Bedbugs Bite

Bedbugs were common in the United States before World War II. With improvements in hygiene, they vanished from our landscape. Like bell-bottoms, alligator shirts and other things best left extinct, these bugs have made a comeback in the United States Bedbugs are brown, flat and about a quarter of an inch long. They hide in crevices like mattresses, box springs and headboards. Inspect your hotel bed to see any evidence of these creatures, and notify management if you see them. If you don't see the bugs themselves, a sign of heavy infestation is dark spotting and rusty or red spots on sheets (it's the dried excrement from the bugs). If the infestation is heavy, you might smell a sweetish yet "buggy" odor. If you get a sweet-smelling room, request a new one.

PART III

Next-Generation Germ Freaks

Kids: Germs Only a Mother Could Love

"As a mom to two kids—a three-year-old and a one-year-old—I cannot believe how clueless people are. I was at a birthday party and someone asked to hold my son. She passed him around to three other people—none of whom I knew. They got right in his face and jiggled him on their knees. After nursing my son through that cold, I don't let strangers pick up my kids."

GERM FREAK MOM

One day it will happen. You won't need to record it in a scrapbook because it will be brandished in your memory forever. It's not the first tooth or the first step or even the first word. It's the first time your baby licks a Cheerio off the floor, lodges his finger up his playmate's nose, or declares with visual in hand, "Look, Mommy, dog-doo is squishy!"

You will learn, through gritted teeth and goopy hands, that parenting is the hardest job in the world, particularly for Germ Freaks. No matter how skilled you are at the task, it's a complete waste of time to attempt proper germ avoidance execution until your kid turns ten (later if you have a boy). Just *try* to be the germ barrier between a houseful of relatives (incoming, incoming!) who flew 1,500 miles (on a germy plane, no less!) to hold the first grandchild. Just try stopping a toddler who's practicing his counting skills by touching every surface in a public bathroom.

You need to learn to walk the line between protecting your child and raising the next Howard Hughes (although he did lead a very interesting life and was, after all, a billionaire). And this is why your motto—for the next few years anyway—will need to shift from "Achoo onto others as you would have them achoo onto you" to "Cringe and bear it." Trust me, it can be done (maybe not perfectly) with a lot of deep breaths . . . and a diaper bag full of wipes.

No matter what kind of parenting expert you follow—Dr. Spock, Dr. Sears or Dr. Seuss—there's one thing every good parent has in common: No parent likes to see their child sick. But it will happen, and it is a natural development in the grand scheme of things. But my question is: What's the rush? They have their whole lives to get germy.

Beware RSP

Since my twins were born seven weeks premature, and in October, the doctor warned us to be careful during the upcoming cold and flu season so that they didn't catch a potentially fatal disease called respiratory syncytial virus, or RSV. But what she forgot to mention was even worse—RSP (Really Stupid People).

If you're a parent, it's your job to protect your child from RSP, whether it's the onlooker who tries to pick up your newborn baby without asking, or the teenager, years down the road, who offers your preteen a beer. There are a lot of RSPs in the world, and you must be prepared to cut them off at the pass.

Because my kids were twins, they got a lot of attention. Every time we went for a walk, to a restaurant, or to the store, people would come up and ask, "Are they twins?" We met many truly sweet people, but we also encountered a lot of touchers. These complete strangers would come up and touch them on their fingers (terrible choice!), their faces (terrible choice!) and their toes (phew, much better!). "Are they twins?" Poke, poke. "You must have your hands full." Poke, poke. *Yes, we sure will have our hands full when you give both of them your cold.*

There's just something about a cute little baby that causes many adults to lose boundaries and brain cells. They may be thinking about their own grandchildren who live far away, or perhaps they're smiling because they're retired and you're the sleep-deprived one, not them. But whatever the reason, these people mean well. Try to be nice to them, or at least tactful. To avoid these situations, talk to your spouse before it happens and come up with a game plan. Presenting a united front will make it easier for both of you to try one of the following tactics:

- Wear your baby in a sling against you—this will keep most people from touching him.
- Dress your baby in cotton baby mittens, a hat and socks to reduce the number of touch points (weather permitting).
- Put a blanket or light towel over the stroller so strangers don't even notice her.
- Tell small children (it works for adults, too) that your baby loves to be tickled on his foot. You can then touch his foot and begin reciting "This little piggy . . ."
- Tell people it's your policy not to let anyone except family hold your baby.
- Blame it on your physician. "My physician told me to keep the baby away from all strangers for three months."
- When your child is older and someone wants to pick him up, tell the person that you're teaching your child that it's not okay to let strangers touch him (this is a good message for overall safety, too).
- Teach your kids to always ask a parent first before touching a baby and to stay away from babies if they have a cold.

Germ Etiquette with
Pregnant Women and Newborns

This topic deserves special attention because these two segments of the population don't have the defenses most of us do against things like colds and flu. A pregnant woman, for instance, can't take NyQuil to relieve her cold. Plus she's already bloated, sometimes nauseous (or about to be soon) and unable to sleep due to a bulging belly. Children don't have the proper defenses to eradicate a cold. By defenses I don't mean their immune response: I mean, they haven't learned how to operate their hardware. Until they are two—or maybe even two and a half if they haven't been to toddler enrichment programs—most kids can't blow their noses. Imagine having a raging cold and not being able to blow your nose! This leaves the parents chasing them about the house, struggling to suction out their noses with a near-useless torture device that looks like a turkey baster (really). Even worse, until a child is verbal, which can range from eighteen months to three years, it's difficult to tell if a tot is teething or has an ear infection. So, for the health of the baby and the sanity of the parents, please follow these guidelines:

· Wash your hands when you visit a newborn. Even if the new parents aren't Germ Freaks, what can it hurt?

· If you must touch a newborn or a baby, touch their feet, not their fingers or their face.

- Don't kiss a baby or toddler on the mouth—you can give a toddler just as much love (even more) with a big bear hug, and a kiss on the head or cheek works fine.
- If you're sick, stay away from newborns and pregnant women.
- Don't feed babies or toddlers (even worse than the germ factor is the choking hazard).
- If a woman is pregnant, don't rub her belly (this has nothing to do with germs; it's just very annoying).

"I have one-year-old twins.
My husband and I try to tell people the tactful way to please refrain from picking them up. They inevitably come back with something like: 'Oh, don't worry, I have children of my own,' or 'It's alright, I'm a grandma myself.'
What difference does that make?
You could be a nana with shingles."

ANOTHER GERM FREAK MOM
(THERE ARE MILLIONS OF US.)

When You Don't Want to Keep Up with the Joneses: Keeping Germs at Bay in Your House

- If you're not breast-feeding, check with your pediatrician about sterilizing bottles and pacifiers.
- Ask all visitors to wash their hands before touching the baby; make a habit of washing your hands when you come in the house and at other appropriate times.
- Regularly clean toys with nontoxic cleaners like hydrogen peroxide or soap and water.
- If your child has had a bad cold or flu, disinfect toys with a mild bleach solution or a disinfecting spray. Rinse them thoroughly.
- As soon as your child is old enough, teach proper hand washing and germ etiquette. Make it fun, and don't be obsessive about it.
- Teach kids to wash their hands for twenty seconds, singing the "ABC Song" to be sure.
- Teach your kids to cough or sneeze into their elbow and to not touch their nose, eyes or mouth (don't expect full, or even half compliance).

A Germ Freak's ✓ GOTTA HAVE IT?

The **Germ Doctor Nursery Product Sanitizer** sanitizes baby's toys in just twenty-one minutes. It uses dry heat, not chemicals, to kill germs and bacteria including staph, E. coli and salmonella. *www.onestepahead.com.*

Kid-Friendly Germ Info

Wash Your Hands. A great book for toddlers by Tony Ross.

Germs. A fun book for kids four to eight, looking at life from the germs' perspective by Ross Collins.

Germs on Their Fingers. A bilingual (English/Spanish) book for ages nine to twelve by Wendy Wakefield Ferrin.

Achoo: The Most Interesting Book You'll Ever Read About Germs. True to its title, a really cool book about germs for kids and their parents by Trudee Romanek.

www.GermsontheRun.com promotes hand washing through fun activities.

www.henrythehand.com. A character and Web site created by a family physician who wanted to stop the cycle of sickness in his own home when his four kids began day care. The Germ Warfare Kit contains a fluorescent black light that simulates germs on your hands, a spritzer bottle, posters and stickers to help kids become champion hand washers.

Petting Zoos

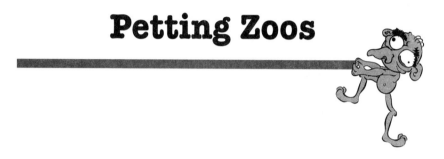

Several outbreaks of serious illness have been associated with petting zoos. In central Florida in 2005, there were fifteen confirmed cases of hemolytic uremic syndrome (HUS), a potentially fatal kidney ailment, from suspected contact at a petting zoo. In 2000, fifty-one people, most of them children, became ill after touching animals at a farm exhibit in Pennsylvania. In Ontario in 1999, more than 150 people developed diarrhea after touching goats at a petting zoo. In all of these cases, E. coli was the cause. After visiting a zoo where Komodo dragons were displayed, twenty people contracted salmonellosis, which can cause diarrhea, meningitis, blood infections and death.

That's right: Our cuddly, furry and feathered friends can carry diseases. While you don't have to avoid zoos altogether, follow these precautions when you go:

- Tell your kids not to touch their faces after they touch any animals (then watch to see that they don't).
- Wash your children's hands thoroughly after petting animals.
- Don't use baby wipes in place of hand washing; these do not kill germs.
- Hand sanitizers may be used as a last resort if no running water is available, but only as a last resort.
- Check out the layout of the zoo: Eat your lunch before your children have touched any animals.
- Don't drink unpasteurized milk or cider if offered at local farms.
- Don't bring pacifiers; if one drops, don't let a child have it back before you disinfect it. Better yet, throw it out.
- Call ahead and make sure the petting zoo is certified by the U.S. Department of Agriculture. If a zoo is USDA certified, it means that the facility meets government standards for the proper care of their animals.
- If your child's school is planning a trip to a zoo, contact the principal to make sure the teachers stress proper hygiene.
- Think twice about hiring a mobile petting zoo for Junior's first birthday extravaganza: Do you want to be known as the mom who got everyone sick? Better to pin the tail on a paper donkey—it's cheaper, too.
- Visit the doctor if you or your child fall ill within three days to two weeks after a trip to the zoo.

Ball Pits

"We went to one of these birthday
affairs at a play center for a boy's first birthday.
I saw my son running to the ball pit with a few
other kids in it. I thought, *No . . . not the
ball pit . . .* As I ran to get him, the ball was in
his mouth. Two days later he was sick."

YET ANOTHER GERM FREAK MOM
(WE'RE EVERYWHERE!)

We've all heard the urban legends about hypodermic needles and rats in the ball pits. These stories have been exaggerated, but the truth is that ball pits are very germy. While some experts say they are no worse than letting your kids play any other place where kids congregate, two leading experts—and many moms—disagree.

Explains Charles Gerba, Ph.D., "These ball pits, especially enclosed in restaurants, are places where parents go to have a burger and throw their kids in there for an hour. It's a haven for little kids ages two to five, some of whom don't have the same sanitary habits as you do. You almost always find E. coli in these pits."

Philip Tierno, Ph.D., states emphatically, "These are not good places for children to cavort."

The only tip for ball pits: **Avoid them.**

Day Care

"As a preschool teacher I see parents
dropping sick kids off all the time. Many times
we have had kids spilling the beans. They'll say,
'I throwed-ed up this morning.' Then we call the
parents to take them home, but it's too late
because they've already touched everything."

PRESCHOOL TEACHER AND GERM FREAK

It's a simple but unsettling fact: Your kids will get sick
more if they attend day care. While the theories abound as to
whether this is better or worse for them in the long run, it doesn't
help you now when you need to deal with what feels like an
onslaught of illness. Take heart in knowing that the older they get,

the less they will be sick. Here are some things you can look for when choosing a center:

- Do they have a hand washing and toilet training policy? Do they teach hygiene habits as part of their day-to-day routine? Ask if they would incorporate a lesson or two devoted to germs. (See *www.germsontherun.com* for ideas.)
- Does your child come home with a diaper rash or get frequent diarrhea? This could indicate improper hygiene.
- Do they have a strict sick policy? Unfortunately, there's not a lot you can do. With many childhood diseases, kids are contagious before they show symptoms.
- How often does the staff clean common areas and shared toys that get mouthed during the day? (It should be daily.) How often do they wash the sleeping mats? (This should be at least weekly.)
- Do they wear gloves or take any measures to reduce infection when changing diapers and wiping noses?
- Is the day care carpeted? While carpets are comfy, they trap germs and are harder to clean than hard surfaces.
- Does the bathroom have adequate soap and water? Paper towels within children's reach?

In a study of 341 children's day care centers, infrequent washing of children's or providers' hands after nose wiping, after diapering, before meals, and before food preparation was "spectacularly" associated with a higher frequency of illness.

- Is the diaper changing area separate from the main area or food prep area?
- Is the food prep area clean? Is one person in charge of food prep? (This cuts down the chances of infection.)

If your child is getting frequent colds or other illnesses, it's not necessarily an indication that the center isn't clean; it could simply be a reflection of outbreaks that are happening in the community. If you feel something is amiss, talk to your pediatrician to ensure your child's immunity is not compromised by lack of sleep or nutrients. Talk to other mothers whose kids are in day care and not in day care to see if their kids are getting sick too. Investigate other day care centers to see if a switch is in order. Plan ahead for emergencies and see if there is a local nanny service or a relative who could care for your child if you have no sick days left. Perhaps there is a stay-at-home mother you trust who would like some additional income during cold and flu season.

Babies who receive their first course of antibiotics during the first six months of life are 2.5 times more likely than their peers to develop asthma by age seven. Babies who received one round of broad-spectrum antibiotics are also 8.9 times more likely to develop asthma.

Treating Ear Infections:
Don't Rush for the Antibiotics

To treat middle ear infection, the American Academy of Pediatrics (AAP) and the American Academy of Family Physicians (AAFP) guidelines emphasize pain relief over antibiotics. Parents are given the option to let their kids fight the infection on their own for forty-eight hours, before beginning antibiotics.

"The whole purpose of these guidelines was to give people a way to intelligently and safely use this option of observing an ear infection," said Dr. Richard M. Rosenfeld, professor and director of pediatric otolaryngology at Long Island College Hospital in New York City. Rosenfeld served as a consultant to the AAP subcommittee that developed the guidelines.

Treating every ear infection with antibiotics is unnecessary, and can make it more difficult to treat future infections. While untreated bacterial ear infections can lead to serious complications including mastoiditis and meningitis, these complications are rare. Under the guidelines, antibiotics are recommended for any child under two or a child with severe symptoms.

Studies show that antibiotics don't make children feel better in the first twenty-four hours. For pain relief, doctors might recommend ibuprofen, acetaminophen or ear drops.

"I find that a lot of parents aren't in a hurry to give antibiotics and are reassured by knowing that 80% of ear infections are cured by the child alone without any meds," said Dr. Kathi J. Kemper, author of *The Holistic Pediatrician*.

Drug-resistant strains of bacteria are more common among children who have recently been treated with antibiotics stronger than amoxicillin, Septra, erythromycin or Pediazole.

A Germ Freak's ✓GOTTA HAVE IT?

GIANTmicrobes plush germs are fuzzy stuffed replicas of real germs. Each stuffed microbe is an accurate representation of how the germ looks, magnified to about 1 million times the actual size. Educational Innovations currently offers the flu, the common cold, streptococcus bacteria (sore throat) and flesh-eating bacteria. Each one comes with an information card about the real-life germ. Contact *www.teachersource.com*.

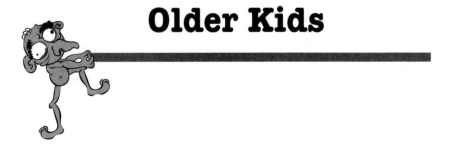

Older Kids

During the course of one year, American children have about six to ten colds; adults average two to four, although women slightly more.

Philip Tierno, Ph.D., joined a group of mothers and kids ages one to four in the suburbs of Long Island, New York. They collected thirty-four germ specimens from everyday things, including the kitchen table, a swing set, an infant walker, toys, a shopping cart handle, a vending machine and school lockers. The heaviest levels of germs occurred as follows:

1. the kitchen table
2. the steering wheel of a children's ride
3. the shopping cart handle

4. the vending machine's coin slot

5. the infant walker

To cut down on your kids' germ load, set up a day each week or biweekly to clean toys, objects and surfaces with nontoxic cleaners like hydrogen peroxide or soap and water.

School

When your child goes off to school, what are the germiest places he'll encounter? According to Dr. Gerba, the three worst areas at one elementary school were the pencil sharpener, the desktop and the water fountain. So pack your kids' lunch each day with a bottle of water and an instant hand sanitizer. While the best situation is that your child goes to the bathroom to wash her hands with soap and water before lunch, it's not always possible. Some kids' schedules are too tight for a bathroom pit stop, and some schools lock up bathrooms unless a monitor is present. In these cases, an alcohol-based sanitizer is better than nothing.

Knox County school officials closed public schools for two days in February 2005 to stop widespread illness of staff and students.

College

Maybe it's the close quarters, the late nights, the lack of home cooking—or all of the above—that make college kids so susceptible to colds, flus and stomach viruses. But every winter several colleges across the country go so far as to suspend operations to stop an outbreak. While each college has its own recommendations for hygiene, the best thing to do is arm your college-bound student with information and supplies.

Collegiate Cold and Flu Season Kit

For the bathroom:

- ❏ Collegiate flip-flops (for bathroom use/hallway walking, see page 178)
- ❏ Cathode Instant Toothbrush Sanitizer (she shouldn't keep her toothbrush in a shared bathroom; sanitize it after every use)
- ❏ Toothbrush carrying case (tuck it safely away after it's sanitized)
- ❏ Pump soap (antibacterial not necessary)

Dorm room:

- ❏ Small HEPA air filter (great for white noise, too)
- ❏ Cell phone (she likely has one already, but if not, no community pay phones to call home, please)
- ❏ First aid kit
- ❏ Airborne/vitamins of choice (vitamins are important, especially if she's not liking the food)

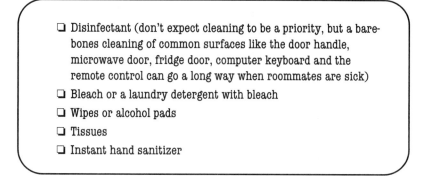

- ❏ Disinfectant (don't expect cleaning to be a priority, but a bare-bones cleaning of common surfaces like the door handle, microwave door, fridge door, computer keyboard and the remote control can go a long way when roommates are sick)
- ❏ Bleach or a laundry detergent with bleach
- ❏ Wipes or alcohol pads
- ❏ Tissues
- ❏ Instant hand sanitizer

Make sure your child knows the symptoms of meningitis and staph infections and is not the type to tough it out instead of seeing the school physician. Not only can an early visit nip something in the bud, it can help identify a potential outbreak. You're paying dearly for the service, so use it.

College freshmen living in dorms are six times more likely to contract meningitis than college students overall; they have the country's highest rate of infection at 5.1 cases per 100,000. Students living on campus had three times the risk of contracting meningitis as students living off campus.

Bacterial meningitis is much more serious than viral meningitis, which is self-limiting and causes flulike symptoms. Symptoms of bacterial meningitis include high fever, stiff neck, severe headache, nausea and a purple rash. It's important for incoming students to be aware of the symptoms, because it's a disease that can kill within a very short time. The disease can be spread by kissing, sharing food or utensils (or keg cup), or inhaling respiratory secretions of an infected person.

A Germ Freak's ✓GOTTA HAVE IT?

Collegiate flip-flops. ToeGoz manufactures collegiate-themed flip-flops in unisex sizes 6 through 13. Colleges include University of Texas, Texas A&M and Arizona State plus fraternities and sororities. *www.flipflopstyle.com.*

Conclusion:
What Goes Around
Comes Around

My family celebrated a recent Thanksgiving at Walt Disney World. There was something going around because everywhere you turned you'd hear someone clearing a throat, stifling a sneeze or coughing. And it wasn't just me who noticed this: My three non–Germ Freak family members noticed too. Before hitting the park, we hit an all-you-can eat, kids-eat-free buffet—a massive germfest for $4.99.

I grabbed my tray and prepared to tackle the smorgasbord—a vat of lumpy oatmeal, shriveled-up sausages and a pile of bagels with no tongs in sight. My husband must have seen my face contorting, despite my best efforts to remain composed. He smirked and plopped a glob of oatmeal on my plate.

"This is just like *Fear Factor* for you, isn't it?"

"No," I told him. "I'd actually prefer pig testicles over this if they were clean."

As I made my way through the line, I saw, out of the corner of my eye, two little kids eating fruit directly out of the bin and going back for more. Didn't their mother teach them any manners? Just as I was about to make a beeline around these germy kids, my husband asked, "How does it feel to see your kids double-dipping?"

I looked closer. Those *were* my kids, foraging their way through the line with their grandmother. He was right: They double-dipped. And since they were twins, they actually quadruple-dipped. The horror! The humility! Had I taught them nothing?!!!

At that moment I realized the enormity of the situation. It was true: What goes around literally does come around . . . and by that I mean germs.

Better safe than sick.

Special Thanks

A special thanks to Charles Gerba, Ph.D., who makes our lives much safer with the tireless work he does. I always enjoyed watching you eek out the germs on television and never thought I'd get the privilege of collaborating with you. Your time and graciousness are very much appreciated as well as the invaluable information you provided to make this book possible.

Thank you to Philip Tierno, Ph.D., and Martin Sloane, for your time and expertise.

Thank you to the many Germ Freaks who shared their tips and experiences with me.

Acknowledgments

A world of thanks to:

Peter Vegso, a generous and gracious man with a big heart, for giving me this opportunity and for building such a special place to work: I won't even hold it against you that the women's room has two germy doors to exit. Bret Witter, an editor extraordinaire and a great boss to boot (did I write this or did you edit it?). I appreciate your hard work spearheading the project and your witty sense of humor; hopefully you've learned eating off the floor is a bad habit . . . even mall cookies. Kathy Grant, the best-accessorized Germ Freak I have the pleasure of knowing: I appreciate your help, your humor and your Lysol every day. To Elisabeth Rinaldi and Amy Hughes for your help and humor. Pat Holdsworth, who could write the advanced *Germ Freak's Guide*, and to Brett Holdsworth for your proofreading and PR skills. Kim Weiss, for your talent in spreading news, not germs. To Lori Golden, Kelly Maragni, Tom Galvin, Sean

Geary and Stephanie Jackson, for your expertise and enthusiasm. Larissa Hise Henoch, for your creativity and the birth of "Icky." Lawna Oldfield, for your talent giving book insides such personality. Mike Briggs, for always getting things done yesterday, with UV coating, die cuts and glitter.

To all of the great people in sales, marketing, production, printing and shipping who did their (typical) outstanding job in making this book, and being fun to work with while doing it.

To Rob, for the "compliment" that inspired the book. I appreciate your support, humor and the computer time to finish this book. I always dreamed of marrying a wonderful person and writing a book: Because of you I'm lucky enough to have done both. Cheryl and Linda, for contributing advice (the book and life) and making me laugh, then and now. My parents, Ted and Joan, for your support and generosity, and for being great grandparents/free babysitters. To my children, for being you. There's nothing better in the world than your big, wet, germy kisses.

Bibliography

Bakalar, Nicholas. *Where the Germs Are: A Scientific Safari.* Hoboken, New Jersey: John Wiley & Sons, Inc., 2003.

Bourdain, Anthony. *Kitchen Confidential: Adventures in the Culinary Underbelly.* New York: HarperCollins, 2000.

Brown, Jack. *Don't Touch That Doorknob: How Germs Can Zap You and How You Can Zap Back.* New York: Warner Books, 2001.

Levy, Elinor, and Mark Fischetti. *The New Killer Diseases: How the Alarming Evolution of Mutant Germs Threatens Us All.* New York: Crown, 2003.

Satin, Morton. *Food Alert: The Ultimate Sourcebook for Food Safety.* (New York: Checkmark Books, 1999.

Thompson, Kimberly, with Debra Bruce Fulgham. *Overkill: How Our Nation's Abuse of Antibiotics and Other Germ Killers is Hurting Your Health and What You Can Do About It.* New York: Rodale, 2002.

Tierno, Philip M. *The Secret Life of Germs: Observations and Lessons from a Microbe Hunter.* New York: Pocket Books, 2001.

Notes

Germ Freak Basics

Farhi, Paul. "In Flu Season the Handshake Loses Favor," *The Washington Post,* December 25, 2004.

"Don't Try to Shake This Man's Hand Until Spring." September 10, 2004. WABC-TV New York.

Gendar, Allison. "Beware the City Travel Bugs! What the News Found and Where We Found It." *New York Daily News.* December 22, 2003.

Lack of hand washing at movie theaters. Phone interview with Charles Gerba, Ph.D., February 11, 2005.

Using disinfecting products. Professor Lester Mitscher. "Anti-Bacterial Cleaners Squash Bugs." *San Francisco Chronicle.* April 26, 2000.

Stuart Levy suggestion to return to tried-and-true cleaners from "War on Bacteria Could Leave Drug-Resistant Strains Unchecked," *Upward Quest Health,* Article 11, July 17, 2000.

Eugene Cole and Nancy Tomes information from article by Jennipher Shaver, "Germ Wars: Experts Wash Away Antibacterial Misconceptions," April 21, 2004, KSBW Channel.com. Tomes, Nancy, "The Making of a Germ Panic, Then and Now," 2000 paper, *The American Journal of Public Health.*

Stuart Levy quote from "War on Bacteria Could Leave Drug-Resistant Strains Unchecked." *Upward Quest Health*, Article 11, July 17, 2000. Presented at the International Conference on Emerging Infectious Diseases, 2000.

The Home Front

de la Cruz, Ralph, "In the Land of the Sick, A Healthy Man Pays the Price," The *Sun-Sentinel*, Tuesday, February 15, 2005.

Charles Gerba, Ph.D., CBS–TV News *48 Hours*, September 28, 2000.

Ann Draughon quote from article, "Cleaned Fruits and Veggies Shouldn't Make Us Sick," in *The Tallahoma News* by Belinda Riddle, February 8, 2005.

Lisa Lachenmayr's quote from "Top 10 Dirtiest Foods," *Men's Health* magazine, May 2004.

At Work

Charles Gerba quote about the survival of the flu virus from *www.surgicenter. online.com*, November 13, 2002.

The Germiest Places at the Workplace. A study by Charles Gerba, Ph.D., conducted by Opinion Research Corporation for Kimberly-Clark Professional, 2003.

Goodman, Ellen, "Sickness Can Cost Jobs," *The Boston Globe*, February 10, 2005.

The Doctor's Office

"Preventing Cold, Flus and Infections," March 16, 1999, *www.drgreene.com*.

The Supermarket

Sloane, Martin. "Dirty Carts: Shame on U.S. Supermarkets!" Part I and II. *www.siteforsavings.com*.

The Public Bathroom

Joe Neumaier, "Monk Comes Clean," *The Age,* January 28, 2004, *www.theage.com.*

Richard Olds quote from "Toilet Seats Get a Bum Rap," by Dru Sefton, Newhouse News Service, 2003.

Charles Ebel quote from "Toilet Seats Get a Bum Rap," by Dru Sefton, Newhouse News Service, 2003.

The Health Club

Gym quote and Where Are the Gym Germs from Philip Tierno on ABC News *Primetime* interview, "Is Your Health Club Unhealthy?" January 13, 2005.

Spas and sauna quote by Philip Tierno, from *The Secret Life of Germs.*

Robert Daum quote from "Superbug MRSA Worries Doctors, Athletes: Drug-Resistant Germ Found in Locker Rooms Can Kill Within Days," ABC News, *Primetime,* January 13, 2005.

David Ropeik quote from "Germs Develop a Deadly Defense," by Emilia Askari, *The Detroit Free Press,* November 12, 2002.

Ron Courson quote from "Superbug MRSA Worries Doctors, Athletes: Drug-Resistant Germ Found in Locker Rooms Can Kill Within Days," ABC News, *Primetime,* January 13, 2005.

Luis-Ostrosky quote. Lerche Davis, Jeanie. "Hilary Swank Kicks Staph Infection: Antibiotics Work Well, but See Doctor When Swelling, Redness Develops." *WebMD Medical News,* January 28, 2005.

Dining Out

Robert Sobsey, "Watching the Inspector," *Reno News and Review,* June 17, 2004 by Brad Bynum.

Philip Tierno quote from phone interview.

Airports and Airplanes

"Another U.S. Airport Travel Hazard—Dirty Hands." Press release, American Society for Microbiology, September 15, 2003, presented at the 43rd Annual Interscience Conference of Antimicrobial Agents and Chemotherapy. Study by Wirthlin Worldwide.

Charles Gerba quote about airplane bathrooms from February 11, 2005 phone interview.

Diana Fairechild quote from "How Safe Is Airline Water?" Letter to the Editor, *The Wall Street Journal,* November 14, 2002.

Timothy McCall quote from *Bottom Line Health,* "Staying Healthy When You Fly," 2002. *www.drmccall.com.*

Cruises

Michael Crye quote from *Florida Today,* December 14, 2003, John McCarthy. "Viruses Become Bane of Cruise Ships."

Next-Generation Germ Freaks

Quotes about ball pits from phone interview with Philip Tierno, and phone interview with Charles Gerba, February 11, 2005.

Rosenfeld and Kemper quotes from "When It Comes to Kids' Ear Infections, Hold the Antibiotic," *HealthDayNews,* February 22, 2005.

The dirtiest places schoolchildren will encounter from a phone interview with Charles Gerba, February 11, 2005.

Resources

Alliance for Prudent Use of Antibiotics, *www.tufts.edu/med/apua*

American Society for Microbiology, *www.microbes.org*

Centers for Disease Control and Prevention, *www.cdc.gov*

For a safer dining experience: Safe Tables Our Priority, S.T.O.P., *www.safetables.org*

For a safer and more pleasant shopping experience: *www.siteforsavings.com*

For a safer trip to a medical office: Timothy B. McCall, M.D., author, *Examining Your Doctor: A Patient's Guide to Avoiding Harmful Medical Care*

For tips on cleaning and decluttering, check out *Cleaning and the Meaning of Life* by Paula Jhung.

For information on nontoxic cleaners check out *www.newdream.org* and *Green Clean: The Enviornmentally Sound Guide to Cleaning Your Home* by Linda Mason Hunter.

For information on safer playgroups go to *www.onlineplaygroup.com*.

About the Authors

Allison Janse is a trade book editor and freelance writer. She feels lucky to call South Florida home because she can justify frequent bulk purchases of sanitizing products as early hurricane preparation. She lives with her husband, who, after ten years of marriage, is showing slight Germ Freak tendencies. Their two children, who they absolutely adore, are proof that being a Germ Freak is not likely a genetic trait.

If you have any Germ Freak horror stories to share, or just want more germ information, contact: *www.germfreaksguide.com.*

Charles Gerba, Ph.D., is an internationally renowned environmental microbiologist who made his reputation a quarter of a century ago by opening scientists' eyes to the dangerous things lurking in our groundwater. His lab created the first test to detect the parasite cryptosporidium in water, changing the way municipalities treat tap water. He is a professor at the University of Arizona where he oversees cutting-edge experiments in the department of Soil, Water & Environmental Science. He has performed thousands of studies on everything from water quality in our homes to urine levels in community pools, from the germs present in airline bathrooms to pathogens in home hot tubs. His quick wit has endeared him to American audiences as Dr. Germ, and he appears regularly on *Good Morning America, Dateline, CNN News* and *60 Minutes* as well as national magazines and newspapers. He lives with his wife in Tuscon, Arizona. Contact Dr. Gerba at: *www.arizona.edu.*